I0066127

Biogenic Amines in Neurotransmission and Human Disease

Edited by Ahmet Uçar

Published in London, United Kingdom

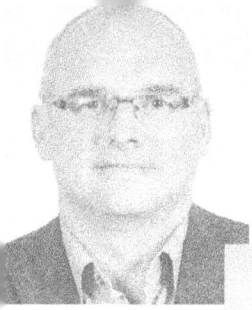
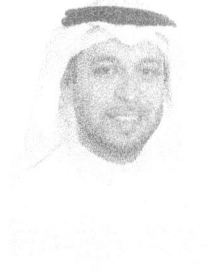
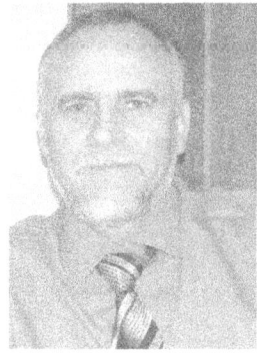
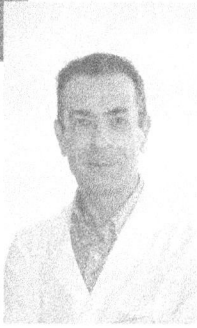
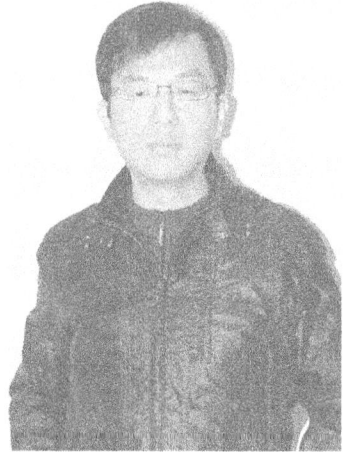
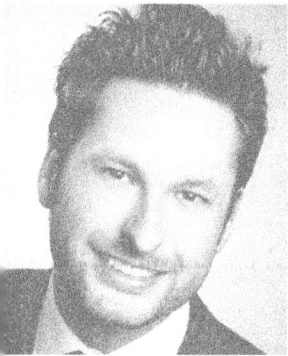
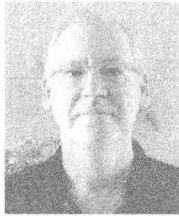

IntechOpen

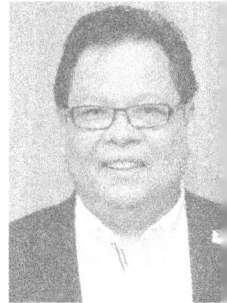
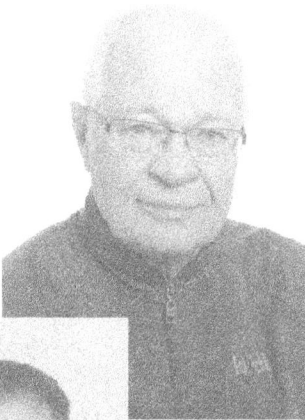
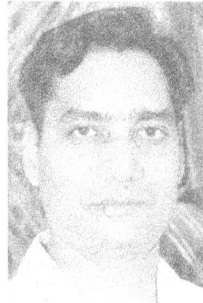
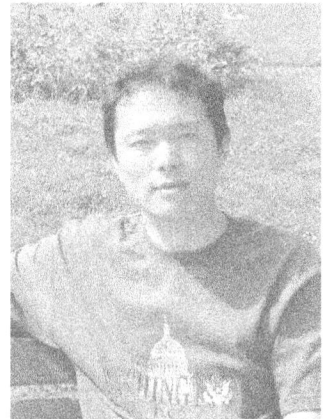
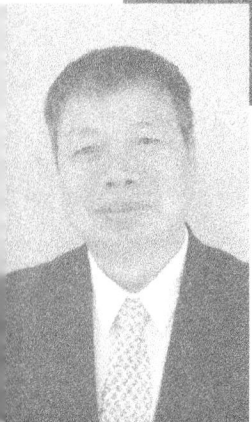
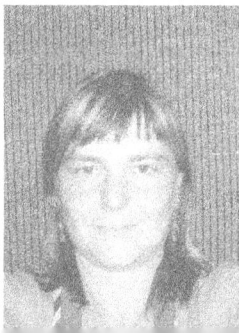

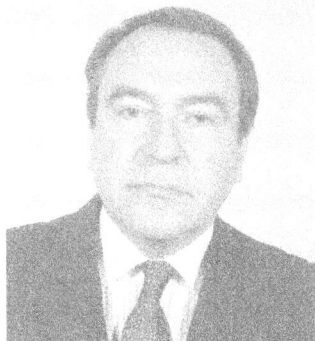

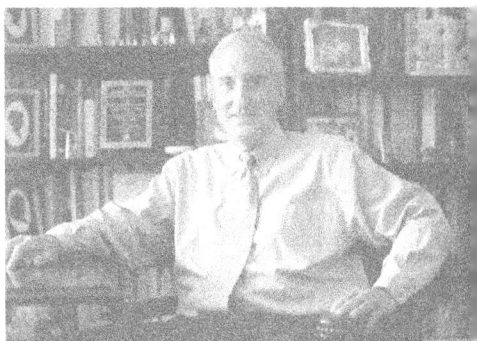

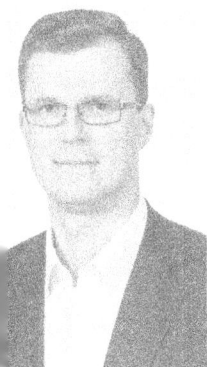

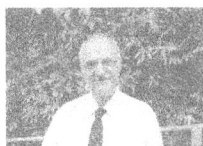

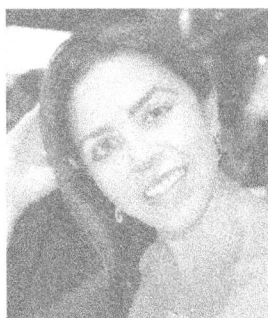

Supporting open minds since 2005

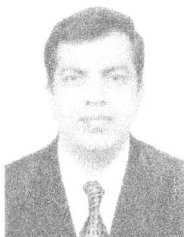

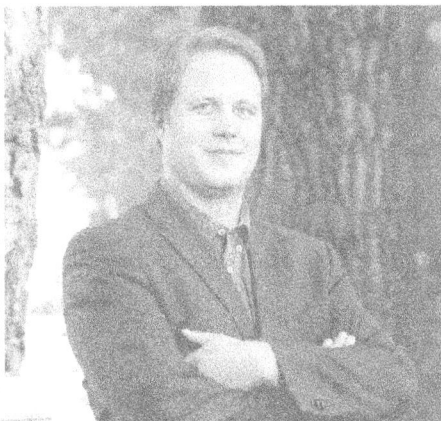

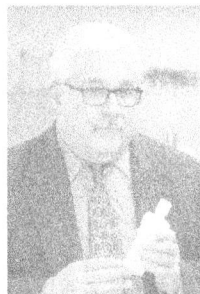

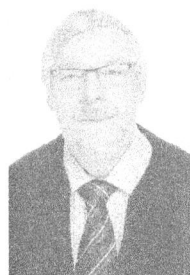

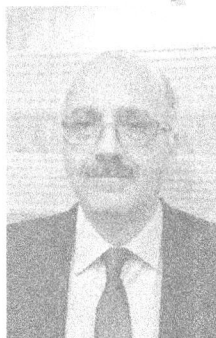

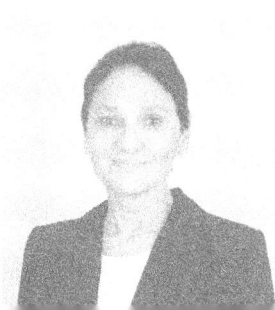

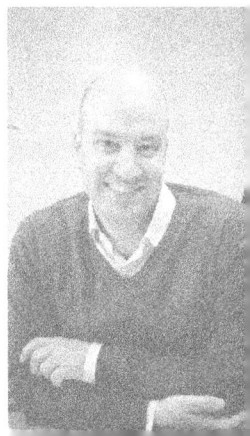

Biogenic Amines in Neurotransmission and Human Disease
http://dx.doi.org/10.5772/intechopen.73738
Edited by Ahmet Uçar

Contributors
Vivek Nambiar, Drisya Rajan, Nobuyuki Yanagihara, Xiaoja Li, Yumiko Toyohira, Noriaki Satoh, Hui Shao, Yasuhiro Nozaki, Fumi Takahashi, Ryo Okada, Hideyuki Kobayashi, Masato Tsutsui, Taizo Kita, Sagrario Martin-Aragon, Paloma Bermejo-Bescós, Pilar González, Juana Benedi, Antonio Rodriguez-Moreno, Pilar Losada-Ruiz, Rafael Falcón.Moya, Ahmet Uçar

© The Editor(s) and the Author(s) 2019
The rights of the editor(s) and the author(s) have been asserted in accordance with the Copyright, Designs and Patents Act 1988. All rights to the book as a whole are reserved by INTECHOPEN LIMITED. The book as a whole (compilation) cannot be reproduced, distributed or used for commercial or non-commercial purposes without INTECHOPEN LIMITED's written permission. Enquiries concerning the use of the book should be directed to INTECHOPEN LIMITED rights and permissions department (permissions@intechopen.com).
Violations are liable to prosecution under the governing Copyright Law.

[(cc) BY]

Individual chapters of this publication are distributed under the terms of the Creative Commons Attribution 3.0 Unported License which permits commercial use, distribution and reproduction of the individual chapters, provided the original author(s) and source publication are appropriately acknowledged. If so indicated, certain images may not be included under the Creative Commons license. In such cases users will need to obtain permission from the license holder to reproduce the material. More details and guidelines concerning content reuse and adaptation can be found at http://www.intechopen.com/copyright-policy.html.

Notice
Statements and opinions expressed in the chapters are these of the individual contributors and not necessarily those of the editors or publisher. No responsibility is accepted for the accuracy of information contained in the published chapters. The publisher assumes no responsibility for any damage or injury to persons or property arising out of the use of any materials, instructions, methods or ideas contained in the book.

First published in London, United Kingdom, 2019 by IntechOpen
IntechOpen is the global imprint of INTECHOPEN LIMITED, registered in England and Wales, registration number: 11086078, 7th floor, 10 Lower Thames Street, London,
EC3R 6AF, United Kingdom
Printed in Croatia

British Library Cataloguing-in-Publication Data
A catalogue record for this book is available from the British Library

Additional hard and PDF copies can be obtained from orders@intechopen.com

Biogenic Amines in Neurotransmission and Human Disease
Edited by Ahmet Uçar
p. cm.
Print ISBN 978-1-83962-863-4
Online ISBN 978-1-83962-864-1
eBook (PDF) ISBN 978-1-83962-865-8

We are IntechOpen,
the world's leading publisher of
Open Access books
Built by scientists, for scientists

4,400+
Open access books available

117,000+
International authors and editors

130M+
Downloads

Our authors are among the

151
Countries delivered to

Top 1%
most cited scientists

12.2%
Contributors from top 500 universities

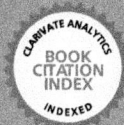

CLARIVATE ANALYTICS
BOOK CITATION INDEX
INDEXED

WEB OF SCIENCE™

Selection of our books indexed in the Book Citation Index
in Web of Science™ Core Collection (BKCI)

Interested in publishing with us?
Contact book.department@intechopen.com

Numbers displayed above are based on latest data collected.
For more information visit www.intechopen.com

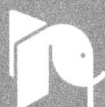

Meet the editor

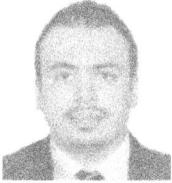

Prior to working at a major university of health sciences, Associate Prof. Ahmet Uçar received his degrees in pediatrics and then in pediatric endocrinology, achieving high honors at the national exams. He has been actively working in the field of pediatric endocrinology and diabetes, and he has contributed significantly to the definition of the characteristics of pubertal variants in children. He successfully completed a thesis on Turner syndrome, which has dramatically increased his interest in and dedication to Turner syndrome ever since. He is an active member of the Turner Syndrome Study Group in Turkey. He is also a member of the Endocrine Society and the European Society of Paediatric Endocrinology.

Contents

Preface

Remarkable advances have been achieved in the elucidation of the mechanisms of involvement of biogenic amines in neurotransmission and human disease. In this book, we briefly review neurotransmission, novel therapeutic options in neurodegeneration, thrombotic tendencies in catecholamine excess states, and the pharmacological potential of plant herbs in dealing with catecholamine associated stress. In the introductory chapter, I summarize the physiology of neurotransmission and describe how biogenic amine excess is associated with human disease, with the example of pheochromocytomas and paragangliomas. In the second chapter, Dr Rodriguez-Moreno describes the latest knowledge on kainate receptors and how they modulate glutamate release in the cerebellum, also presenting some insight on how aberrations in the described pathways relate to human disease. In the third chapter, Prof. Martin-Aragon describes the recent advances in the therapeutic management of neurodegenerative diseases, also giving some insight into homeostatic plasticity, which refers to the capacity of neurons to regulate their own excitability relative to network activity, a compensatory adjustment that occurs over the timescale of days. Therapies to modulate neuronal plasticity to halt neurodegeneration and their related clinical findings have shown much progress in the last decade, with enhanced understanding of neurobiology and molecular genetics that now allow genome editing that has the potential to halt the progress of neurodegeneration. In the fourth chapter, Prof. Nobuyuki presents information on the potential effects of plant herbs in alleviating the stress induced by catecholamine signaling. In the last chapter, the mechanisms regarding thrombotic tendencies in catecholamine excess are covered by Dr Rajan. The last two chapters succinctly describe how catecholamine excess states are associated with derangements in multiple systems in the human body.

I hope this book will serve as a point of reference and source of inspiration for researchers and clinicians interested in addressing issues regarding biogenic amine excess- or deficiency- related diseases in humans.

Ahmet Uçar, MD
Associate Professor,
University of Health Sciences,
Şişli Hamidiye Etfal Education and Research Hospital,
Istanbul, Turkey

Introductory Chapter: Biogenic Amines in Neurotransmission and Human Disease from the Endocrinologist's Perspective

Ahmet Uçar

1. A synopsis of the normal physiology of neurotransmission in man

There are about 10^{11} neurons and 10^{14} synaptic connections in the human brain. The neural circuitry is continuously sculpted in response to experience, modified as we learn and store memories, and irreversibly altered by the gradual loss of neurons and connections as we age [1].

Neuronal signals are transmitted from cell to cell at synapses. When an action potential arrives at the presynaptic site, the depolarization of the membrane opens voltage-gated calcium channels that are clustered in the presynaptic membrane. Calcium influx triggers the release of neurotransmitters which are stored in membrane-enclosed synaptic vesicles and released by exocytosis. The neurotransmitter provokes an electrical change in the postsynaptic cell by binding to and opening transmitter-gated ion channels. After the neurotransmitter is secreted into the synaptic cleft, it is rapidly removed: it is either destroyed by specific enzymes in the synaptic cleft or taken up by the presynaptic nerve terminal or by surrounding glial cells. Reuptake is mediated by a variety of Na^+-dependent neurotransmitter symporters. The cycling of neurotransmitters allows cells to keep up with the high rates of release [1–3].

The chemical or electrical synapses can be excitatory or inhibitory. Excitatory neurotransmitters open cation channels, causing an influx of Na^+ and also Ca^+ in many cases, which reduces the threshold to fire an action potential. Inhibitory neurotransmitters open Cl^- or K^+ channels, thereby making it difficult to depolarize the cell membrane. Depending on the secretion milieu, the type of the receptors they bind to, and the ionic conditions that they encounter, transmitters may be either inhibitory or excitatory. For example, acetylcholine may have inhibitory or excitatory effects depending on the type of the receptor it binds to. Usually glutamate and serotonin are excitatory, whereas γ-aminobutyric acid and glycine are inhibitory [1–4]. All neurotransmitter receptors fall into one of these classes based on their signaling mechanisms:

1. Ionotropic receptors—ion channels present at fast chemical synapses. Example: acetylcholine receptor of skeletal muscle cells is a transmitter-gated ion channel which is opened transiently by acetylcholine released from the nerve terminal at a neuromuscular junction.

2. Metabotropic receptors—also called G protein-coupled receptors. Signaling via is these receptors is somewhat slower, more complex, and longer lasting in its effects. For example: hormones such as parathyroid hormone operate via G protein-coupled receptors [1].

Biogenic amines such as dopamine, norepinephrine, serotonin, and histamine manifest their effects either directly or indirectly via their specified receptors [1].

2. Biogenic amines in human disease

Any dysfunction that occurs in the aforementioned physiological setups in the organism may be associated with a disease state, mostly with neurological consequences, and therapy is aimed at inducing the recovery of the dysfunctional pathway via drugs or, most recently, the gene therapy, which is elaborating ground-breaking results [5].

Disorders of neurotransmission in the human are either due to the lack of synthesis of the neurotransmitter, disordered synapse due to external insults such as trauma, autoimmunity, or impaired or enhanced receptor-ligand interaction at the postsynaptic area. The list of the neurogenerative diseases, the inborn errors of metabolism associated with dysfunctional neurotransmission, is not exhaustive and is discussed elsewhere [6].

From the endocrinologist's perspective, excess of biogenic amines includes many rare endocrine neoplasias such as pheochromocytomas (PHEO) and paragangliomas (PGL). The carcinoid syndrome, a constellation of clinical symptoms of biogenic amine excess particularly of serotonin, is much rarer in clinical practice, and it is usually observed in the context of clinically manifest neuroendocrine tumors, such as midgut carcinoids. In the pediatric patient, these syndromes of *amine excess* are usually associated with hereditary syndromes of endocrine neoplasia, such as von Hippel-Lindau disease and multiple endocrine neoplasia (MEN) type 2 syndrome, whereas sporadic cases are more common in the adult [7]. The diagnosis of *amine excess* states is challenging since single measurement of the culprit molecules via standard laboratory tests is often inconclusive and full of caveats that mandate repeat measurements of the suspected amines and/or their metabolites. Below is a brief description of catecholamine excess related tumors as an example to how *biogenic amine excess* may relate to human disease.

Pheochromocytomas and paragangliomas (PGL) are uncommon neuroendocrine tumors of neural crest origin, with the former being of adrenal medulla origin and the latter originating from sympathetic and parasympathetic system. All functional PHEO/PGL produce and metabolize catecholamines and contain chromaffin tissue, which refers to the brownish black color due to oxidation of catecholamines after staining with chromium salts. Pheochromocytomas comprise the majority of the tumors in the pediatric patient [7].

Dopamine, norepinephrine, and epinephrine are biogenic amines collectively referred to as catecholamines. These neurotransmitters and hormones are involved in regulation of numerous physiological processes and development of neuropsychiatric and cardiovascular diseases. They are synthesized from tyrosine, which is converted to 3,4-dihydroxyphenylalanine (DOPA) by the enzyme tyrosine hydroxylase, the rate-limiting enzyme in catecholamine synthesis. Decarboxylation and hydroxylation of dopa yield dopamine and norepinephrine, respectively. Norepinephrine is then converted to epinephrine via the enzyme phenylethanolamine N-methyltransferase.

The complex actions of norepinephrine and epinephrine are mediated by the G protein-coupled alpha- and beta-adrenergic receptors, whereas dopamine binds to a different class of metabotropic receptors.

The clinical presentation PHEO/PGL is variable. Owing to the neuroendocrine origin, they might co-secrete other hormones that result ectopic hormone excess, such as gigantism due to growth hormone-releasing hormone, hypercalcemia due to parathyroid hormone-related peptide, or secretory diarrhea due to vasoactive intestinal peptide. The clinical symptoms and signs of functional PHEO/PGL also depend on differences in catecholamine secretion and release as individual patient sensitivities to catecholamines. Signs of catecholamine excess include hypertension, headaches, palpitations, diaphoresis (less common in children), orthostatic hypotension, pallor, tremor, and anxiety. Depending on the location of the tumor, nonspecific signs and symptoms include blurred vision, abdominal pain, diarrhea, or behavioral problems/decline in school performance [7].

The diagnosis of excess catecholamine secretion due to PHEO/PGL has been facilitated by the development of assays sensitive to diagnose these entities; measurements of fractionated metanephrine and normetanephrine in plasma and urine are considered the primary diagnostic tests in the initial evaluation of suspected PHEO/PGL. An elevation of metanephrines greater than fourfold above the reference range is considered indicative of a catecholamine secreting tumor [8]. It should be noted that some PGL can be nonfunctional and may be diagnosed incidentally or due to clinical signs and symptoms owing to their anatomical position, as is the case in some paragangliomas of the head neck which arise from parasympathetic ganglia. Catecholamine-secreting tumors may be noradrenergic as in tumors associated with von Hippel-Lindau disease and familial PGL or adrenergic as seen in tumors that arise sporadically or in the context of MEN type 2 and neurofibromatosis type 1. Dopamine-secreting tumors are very rare and typically extra-adrenal succinate dehydrogenase-mediated paragangliomas. Measurement of methoxytyramine may be of help in this context, but the test is not widely available [9]. Chromogranin A is also another effective tumor marker that may correlate with tumor size and malignant potential.

Radiographic studies and in selected cases, molecular genetic testing should be planned once the diagnosis of catecholamine secreting tumor is highly considered. Further information on management of PHEO/PGL is discussed elsewhere [7].

The expanding knowledge on synthesis and function of biogenic amines may pave the path for enhanced medical treatment of disease states of owing to *biogenic amine excess*. Recent studies have also shown that biogenic amines have additional important roles as signaling molecules mediating the function of the "microbiota-brain-gut" axis [10]. The potential role of biogenic amines in this axis is an exciting new area of medicine that awaits for further studies.

Author details

Ahmet Uçar
Health Sciences University, Şişli Hamidiye Etfal Education and Research Hospital, Istanbul, Turkey

*Address all correspondence to: aucar76@yahoo.com

IntechOpen

© 2019 The Author(s). Licensee IntechOpen. This chapter is distributed under the terms of the Creative Commons Attribution License (http://creativecommons.org/licenses/by/3.0), which permits unrestricted use, distribution, and reproduction in any medium, provided the original work is properly cited. [cc] BY

References

[1] Alberts B, Johnson A, Lewis J, et al. Chapter 11. Membrane transport of small molecules and the electrical properties of membranes. In: Molecular Biology of the Cell. Sixth ed. Garland-Norton. 2014. pp. 597-640

[2] Davis GW. Homeostatic control of neural activity: From phenomenology to molecular design. Annual Review of Neuroscience. 2006;**29**:307-323

[3] Jessel TM, Kandel ER. Synaptic transmission: A bidirectional and self-modifiable form of cell-cell communication. Cell. 1993;**72**(Suppl):1-30

[4] Numa S. A molecular view of neurotransmitter receptors and ionic channels. Harvey Lectures. 1987;**83**:121-165

[5] Robert Nussbaum RR, McInnes HF, editors. Willard chapter 13 treatment of genetic disease. In: Thompson and Thompson Genetics in Medicine. 8th ed. Elsevier; 2016. pp. 257-282

[6] Robert Nussbaum RR, McInnes HF, editors. Willard, chapter 12. The molecular, biochemical and cellular basis of genetic disease. In: Thompson and Thompson Genetics in Medicine. 8th ed. Elsevier; 2016. pp. 215-257

[7] Waguespack SG, Ying AK. Chapter 14: Pheochromocytomas and multiple endocrine neoplasia syndromes. In: Mark A, editor. Pediatric Endocrinology. 4th ed. Elsevier Saunders, Sperling; 2014. pp. 533-568

[8] Eisenhofer G, Goldstein DS, Walter MM, et al. Biochemical diagnosis of pheochromocytoma: How to distinguish true- from false-positive test results. The Journal of Clinical Endocrinology and Metabolism. 2003;**88**:2656-2666

[9] Eisenhofer G, Goldstein D, Sullivan P, et al. Biochemical and clinical manifestations of dopamine-producing paragangliomas: Utility of plasma methoxytyramine. The Journal of Clinical Endocrinology and Metabolism. 2005;**90**:2068-2075

[10] Sudo N. Biogenic amines: Signals between commensal microbiota and gut physiology. Frontiers in Endocrinology. 2019;**10**:504. DOI: 10.3389/fendo.2019.00504

Chapter 2

Kainate Receptors Modulating Glutamate Release in the Cerebellum

Pilar Losada-Ruiz, Rafael Falcón-Moya
and Antonio Rodríguez-Moreno

Abstract

Glutamate receptors of the kainate type (Kainate receptors, KARs), are mediators of ionotropic postsynaptic synaptic transmission, as well as presynaptic modulators of neurotransmitter release where they show both ionotropic and metabotropic actions regulating glutamate and γ-aminobutiric acid (GABA) release. The mechanisms underlying these modulatory roles are starting to be understood at some brain regions. Here we review the KARs roles and mechanisms involved in the modulation of glutamate release in the cerebellum at parallel fibers (PF)-Purkinje Cells (PuC) synapses. KARs activation mediate a biphasic effect on glutamate release at this synapse, with low kainate (KA) concentrations mediating a facilitation of glutamate release and higher KA concentrations mediating a depression of glutamate release. KA-mediated facilitation is prevented by antagonizing KARs, by inhibition of PKA or stimulation of adenylyl cyclase (AC), by blocking Ca^{2+} permeant KARs, by depleting intracellular Ca^{2+} stores and by blocking calmodulin. Thus, at cerebellar parallel fiber-Purkinje cell synapses, presynaptic KARs mediate glutamate release facilitation through Ca^{2+}-calmodulin dependent activation of adenylyl cyclase/cAMP/protein kinase A signaling. KAR-mediated depression of glutamate release involves the AC/cAMP/PKA pathway as for facilitation but not Ca^{2+}-calmodulin, being in this case AC activated by a Gi/o protein to mediate a depression of glutamate release.

Keywords: cerebellum, KARs, glutamate release, presynaptic, PKA, adenylate cyclase, Ca^{2+} calmodulin

1. Introduction

Glutamate is the most abundant excitatory neurotransmitter in the central nervous system (CNS) of mammals. Glutamate mediates its actions by activating glutamate receptors. These receptors participate in normal synaptic transmission at different synapses, in plasticity processes as long-term potentiation (LTP) and long-term depression (LTD) that are considered the cellular and molecular correlation of memory and learning processes and in synaptogenesis and neuronal maturation and, additionally, failure in the functioning of this system can be the origin of some types of epilepsy and may contribute to the development of CNS disorders such as

Alzheimer's disease, Huntington's Korea, amyotrophic lateral sclerosis, Parkinson's disease, hypoglycemia, or cerebral ischemia [1–3].

Glutamate receptors are classically divided into two large families: ionotropic and metabotropic. Ionotropic glutamate receptors (iGluRs) participate in rapid neurotransmission in the nervous system; these ionotropic receptors are classified into three types depending on the agonist that activates them with higher affinity: N-methyl-D-aspartic acid (NMDA) receptors (NMDARs), α-amino-3-hydroxy-5-methyl-4-isoxazolepropionic acid (AMPA) receptors (AMPARs), and kainate receptors (KARs). These receptors form a channel with different selectivity depending on their subunit composition, all of them being permeable to Na^+ and K^+ and, additionally, NMDARs are permeable to Ca^{2+} been some AMPARs and KARs also permeable to Ca^{2+} depending on subunit composition. They are integral membrane proteins, formed by four subunits (tetramers), being homomers or heteromers [1, 2].

Metabotropic glutamate receptors (mGluRs), which participate also in neurotransmission, are coupled to G proteins and are divided into eight types (mGluR 1–8) and three groups of receptors: group I mGluRs includes mGluR1 and mGluR5 receptors. These receptors are positively coupled to phospholipase C (PLC), which facilitates the conversion of inositol diphosphate (PIP2) to diacylglycerol (DAG) and inositol triphosphate (IP3). DAG activates protein kinase C (PKC) that phosphorylates different substrates and IP3 causes numerous intracellular effects, including the facilitation of Ca^{2+} release from intracellular stores. Group II mGluRs includes mGluR2 and mGluR3 receptors. These receptors are negatively coupled to adenylate cyclase-mediated AMPc formation, and group III mGluRs includes mGluR4, mGluR6, mGluR7, and mGluR8 receptors. These receptors are negatively coupled to the formation of AMPc mediated by adenylate cyclase [4].

1.1 Kainate receptors

Kainate (KA) is a potent neurotoxin derived from the alga *Digenea simplex*. The word "Kainic" is derived from the Japanese "Kaininso" ("Makuri"), which means "the ghost of the sea," and it is an agonist for both KARs and AMPARs (in the same way that the AMPARs agonist AMPA may activate KARs). Kainate is classically known for its potent epileptogenic actions [5, 6].

KA (and other agonists) activates KARs that are tetramers that resulted from different combinations of five subunits called GluK1, GluK2, GluK3, GluK4, and GluK5 (formerly known as GluR5, GluR6, GluR7 and KA1, and KA2, respectively). Of these subunits, GluK1 and GluK3 may form homomeric or heteromeric functional receptors, while GluK4 and GluK5 may only participate in functional receptors when associated with any of the GluK1, GluK2, or GluK3 subunits, but they do not combine with subunits of AMPARs [1, 7, 8].

KARs have been described in different invertebrates such as nematodes and flies [9, 10] and in different species of vertebrates such as amphibia, fish, and birds [11–13] in addition to mammals. In mammals, KARs have been observed virtually throughout the entire nervous system, although their subcellular location has not been yet fully determined. KARs are widely distributed throughout the CNS and found in the main cells and interneurons of the hippocampus, lateral amygdala, dorsal root ganglia, bipolar cells of the retina, cerebral cortex, and the cerebellum [14, 15].

The lack of knowledge about these receptors compared to other glutamatergic receptors (AMPARs or NMDARs) has been due to the lack of good agonist and antagonist for receptors with particular subunit compositions and to the absence of specific antibodies for the different subunits of KARs, being therefore a significant limitation when exploring the distribution of these receptors. However, by using in situ hybridization techniques, it has been observed that the cells that present a significant expression of the kainate-type subunits GluK1, GluK2, GluK3, and GluK5 are distributed throughout the CNS, including nucleus striatum, hippocampus, cortex, and cerebellum [16]. Likewise, there is a high expression of the GluK4 subunit in the CA3 region of the hippocampus, as well as in the granular neurons of the dentate gyrus. The messenger of the GluK5 subunit, on the other hand, appears more abundantly and more extensively than that of the GluK4 subunit or those of the other subunits [15]. Because the in situ hybridization technique is informative and cannot reveal the subcellular distribution of a specific subunit, and because of pharmacological limitations, there is still much to know about the subcellular location and physiology of these receptors.

Kainate-type glutamate receptors are well established mediators of canonical, ionotropic postsynaptic synaptic transmission and, presynaptically, have a modulatory role in regulating neurotransmitter release. In the latter regard, KARs have been shown to have a noncanonical metabotropic capacity, whereby they affect the control of both glutamate and GABA release, for review see [15, 17–22]. At some excitatory glutamatergic synapses, KARs' activation can actually effect biphasic modulation, where low agonist concentrations facilitate glutamate release, while high concentrations decrease the release of the neurotransmitter, for review see [17, 18]. Mechanistic details of how this is achieved are subject of investigation and, indeed, the subcellular location of KARs responsible for presynaptic modulation remains contentious. Different roles of KARs in plasticity have also been described either in LTP or LTD, see [23] for a review of the role of KARs in plasticity.

As other glutamate receptors, KARs are directly or indirectly involved in different diseases, alterations of the nervous system and neurodegeneration and cell death processes. As previously indicated, KA is a potent neurotoxin that directly induces epilepsy and is used as a temporal lobe epilepsy model [5, 6]. Several lines of research indicate that KA directly activating KARs is involved in excitatory and inhibitory imbalances associated with epilepsy. The use of animal models for epilepsy through the use of KA injections has allowed to reproduce in great detail the symptoms observed in humans. The majority of studies of KARs' involvement in epilepsy have studied acute KA-induced seizures [24–27]. The best demonstrations of a mechanism for KARs' involvement in acute epilepsy come from studies of inhibition of GABA release by the activation of presynaptic KA receptors at interneuron-CA1 hippocampal synapses [24, 28, 29]. In chronic epilepsy, a role of KARs has been demonstrated at hippocampal mossy fibers making aberrant synapses onto granule cells of dentate gyrus expressing high number of KARs [30–32] reviewed in [6, 33]. In humans, genetic studies of members of a family affected by idiopathic juvenile absence epilepsy found elevated levels of Grik1 polymorphisms [34], and in TLE patients, GluK1 subunit containing KARs' increased levels have also been found [35]. In clinical studies, NS1209 (an AMPA/KARs' antagonist) has been found to decrease epileptic symptoms [36].

Different studies of neurotoxicity clearly indicate that KARs might be important targets for neuroprotection in neurons and glial cells. The mechanism by which KARs produce excitotoxicity and neuronal cell death is not well understood mainly because of the limitations in appropriate pharmacological tools. Toxicity of KARs involved in multiple sclerosis has also been found onto oligodendrocytes and myelin related to [37, 38], and damage has also been found at axonal levels, where AMPA/KARs' antagonists prevent it [39]. Interestingly, KARs have also been involved in pain. They are present at dorsal roots activating nociceptors, actually there are clinical trials using KARs' antagonists to try to prevent pain showing some levels of analgesia [36]. Additionally, KARs have been involved in ischemia [40, 41], migraine pain [36], Alzheimer's disease [42], Parkinson's disease [43, 44], Huntington's Chorea [45–47], Schizophrenia [48, 49], depression [50], bipolar disorder [51, 52], mental retardation [53], and autism [54, 55] as reviewed in [56]. In general, antagonists of KARs containing particular subunits might be good targets to ameliorate symptoms or treat different CNS diseases and alterations.

2. KARs in the cerebellum

As indicated above, KARs are expressed in the cerebellar cortex [57–59]. As known, the cerebellum participates in the modulation of movement by modifying the activity patterns of motor neurons. Structurally, the cerebellum is composed of the laminar cerebellar cortex and the deep cerebellar nuclei and has five types of cells: Purkinje, stellate, basket, Golgi, and granule cells. Purkinje cells (PuC) are aligned in front of each other. Their dendritic trees form two 2-dimensional layers through which parallel fibers from the mossy fibers located in the granular layer pass. These parallel fibers (PF) establish excitatory synapses between granular cells and the spines of the PCs dendrites as well as the climbing fibers (CF, originating from the inferior olivary nucleus) with the nearby dendrites and the cellular soma. The parallel fibers pass orthogonally through the dendritic tree of the Purkinje neuron. Up to 200,000 PF form a synapse with a single PuC. Each PuC receives up to 500 synapses of CF, all originated from a single CF. Both basket cells and stellate cells provide an inhibitory (GABAergic) entry to the PuC, with cells in the basket synapse to the initial segment of the PuC axon, and stellate cells to the dendrites [60, 61].

Presynaptic KARs participate in plasticity in the cerebellum where PF synapses onto PuCs mediate a form of LTD that is affected by the paired activation of CFs [62], **Table 1**; of these two types of fibers (PF and CF synapsing onto the same cells (PC), only PF have presynaptic KARs [62], similar to other brain regions as somatosensory and visual cortices in which fibers containing and noncontaining presynaptic ionotropic glutamate receptors synapse onto the same postsynaptic cell and induce LTD [63–69]. The exact role and action mechanism of KARs mediating LTD in the cerebellum are not well known yet and await further investigation.

The proper cerebellum development depends on a precise coordinated sequence of postnatal events, some of which are mediated by glutamate receptors. For example, NMDA receptors have been implicated in the migration of granular cells [70] and in the synaptic pruning of climbing fibers [71]. Although it has recently been shown that KARs are involved in synaptic transmission, little is known about their role in development. However, the expression of kainate-type glutamate receptor subunits in immature granule cells of the outer germinal layer of the developing cerebellum suggests that KARs may also have a role in neuronal maturation. Throughout the maturation process of the cerebellum, the quantity, composition, and function of KARs vary. Initially, cerebellar granular cells have a minimal amount of AMPARs in the postnatal period compared to KARs, which are predominant in immature granule cells. Different studies have shown that KARs composed of subunits GluK1, GluK2, and GluK5 predominate, and over the period of development, an increase in the number of KARs is observed and once the adult stage is reached, the number of KARs containing GluK1 subunits suffers a reduction in their expression in the granular layer, while the GluK2 and GluK5 remain constant, in contrast to AMPARs that increase their number, constituting a very notable majority compared to KARs.

KARs' activation	High concentrations of kainate	Depression of glutamatergic synaptic transmission	Delaney and Jahr [86]
	Low concentrations of kainate	Facilitation of glutamatergic synaptic synaptic transmission	Falcón-Moya et al. [80]
	Ionic imbalance	Calcification	Korf and Postema [78]
	Increase in Ca^{2+}	Neurodegeneration	
	Nodular cerebellum lesion Putrescine increase Histological damage	Ataxia	Maiti et al. [72] de Vera et al. [73] Yamaguchi et al. [74] Andoh et al. [75]
Parallel fibers paired with postsynaptic depolarization	Presynaptic KARs' activation	Long-term depression	Crépel [62]
Increase of GluR6 and GluK2 receptors	Reduction of GABAergic activity	Schizophrenia	Harrison et al. [76] Bullock et al. [77]

Table 1.
KARs' actions in the cerebellum.

All of these findings suggest that KARs have an important role in the development process of the cerebellum. Some indications suggest that GluK1-containing KARs participate in cerebellar development in the beginning of the differentiation of granular cells.

Additionally, KARs have been involved in some brain alterations in the cerebellum and a direct relationship exists between KA injection and cerebellar ataxia. Thus, the cerebellum is an important target to study functions of KARs and its possible role causing ataxia [72–75]. Furthermore, in patients with schizophrenia, an increase in KARs containing GluR6 and K2 subunits is observed, which would mediate a reduction in GABAergic transmission [76, 77]. In neurodegeneration, KARs may have a role in calcification of the brain tissue as it has been found that local application of KA in some areas of the cerebellum produces changes in different ion levels, highly increasing Ca^{2+} levels for more than 8 weeks, which mediate calcification [78] (**Table 1**). KARs have been described as producing increases in intracellular calcium [79, 80] and seems to signal increasing intracellular calcium without putting the cell at risk due to excitotoxicity, due to its low conductance in contrast to AMPARs. Due to the lack of knowledge on the subject, further exploration is necessary to determine the KARs' role in cerebellum development and cerebellar alterations.

2.1 KARs modulating glutamate release in the cerebellum: a biphasic effect

KARs are known to be expressed in the cerebellar cortex in the axons of cerebellar granule cells that form PF and make excitatory synapses with PuC [58]. Messenger RNA transcripts encoding for different KAR subunits and functional expression of KAR subtypes have been reported [81–84]. Biophysical studies with single-channel recording have shown GluK1 activity [85], suggesting these KARs are Ca^{2+} permeable. A biphasic action of KARs, activated by the agonist domoate, has been shown previously at PF-PuC synapse, with low agonist concentrations, facilitating synaptic transmission and higher concentrations depressing synaptic transmission [86] in agreement with what has been found in the hippocampus [87–89], cortex [90], amygdala [91], and the thalamus [92]. EPSC trial-to-trial fluctuation analysis, failure rates, as well as paired-pulse ratios have shown that these facilitatory and depressive actions of KARs in the cerebellum are mediated by presynaptic KARs [80]. However, the precise mechanism of action by which KARs mediate potentiation (and depression) of synaptic transmission at PF-PuC synapses has remained elusive until very recently [80] (**Table 1**).

2.1.1 Action mechanism for KARs-mediated facilitation of glutamate release at cerebellar PF-PuC synapses

We have recently demonstrated that the effect of the KARs' activation in this synapse requires protein kinase A (PKA) activation, since the inhibition of this protein by cAMP-Rp suppresses the effect of KA in glutamate release [80], in agreement with previous studies in hippocampus and cortex [87–89]. This congruence between mechanisms at different synapses has also been seen through the inhibition of PKA using H-89, which eliminates KARs-mediated facilitation of glutamate release. Similarly, the direct activation of AC (adenylyl cyclase) using forskolin caused an elimination of facilitation when KARs were activated by KA (with NMDARs and AMPARs blocked). These data indicate that a signaling mediated by AC/cAMP/PKA supports the facilitation of the modulation of synaptic transmission/glutamate release in these cerebellar synapses (**Figures 1–3**).

As observed in other synapses, Ca^{2+} seems to play a fundamental role in facilitating glutamate release at PF-PuC synapses. By blocking calcium-permeable KARs by the selective inhibitor philanthotoxin, KAR-mediated synaptic facilitation of glutamate release was prevented, indicating that there is a strict requirement for external Ca^{2+} entry through KARs to support the facilitation effect observed on glutamate release, indicating that KARs mediating the facilitation of glutamate release are calcium permeable [80].

Additionally, as has been reported at hippocampal synapses, the depletion of intracellular Ca^{2+} stores by a treatment with thapsigargin (a noncompetitive calcium inhibitor of the sarcoplasmic reticulum ATPase) eliminates the facilitation of glutamate release mediated by KARs' activation. The same result was found when selectively inhibiting Ca^{2+}-induced calcium release by using ryanodine, indicating that the entry of Ca^{2+} via KARs induces a mobilization of Ca^{2+} from the intraterminal Ca^{2+} reserves to mediate the increase in glutamate release observed [80].

Furthermore, it has been observed that the facilitation of glutamate release mediated by the activation of KARs is sensitive to calmodulin inhibitors. Previous studies showed that the increase of cytosolic calcium levels activates Ca^{2+} dependent on AC present in the terminals of parallel fibers. Through treatment with the calmodulin inhibitors, W-7 and calmidazolium, it has been recently shown [80] that the inhibition of calcium-calmodulin function prevents KAR-mediated presynaptic facilitation of glutamate release in cerebellar slices, supporting the hypothesis that after KAR activation and cytosolic elevation of Ca^{2+}, a calmodulin-dependent calcium coupling activates AC, which subsequently activates the AC/cAMP/PKA pathway, thus promoting synaptic facilitation through an increase in neurotransmitter release at PF-PuC synapses [80].

2.1.2 Action mechanism for KARs-mediated depression of glutamate release at cerebellar PF-PuC synapses

Recently, in the same study discussed in the previous section [80], a transient synaptic depression of glutamate release with high concentrations of KA (3 µM)

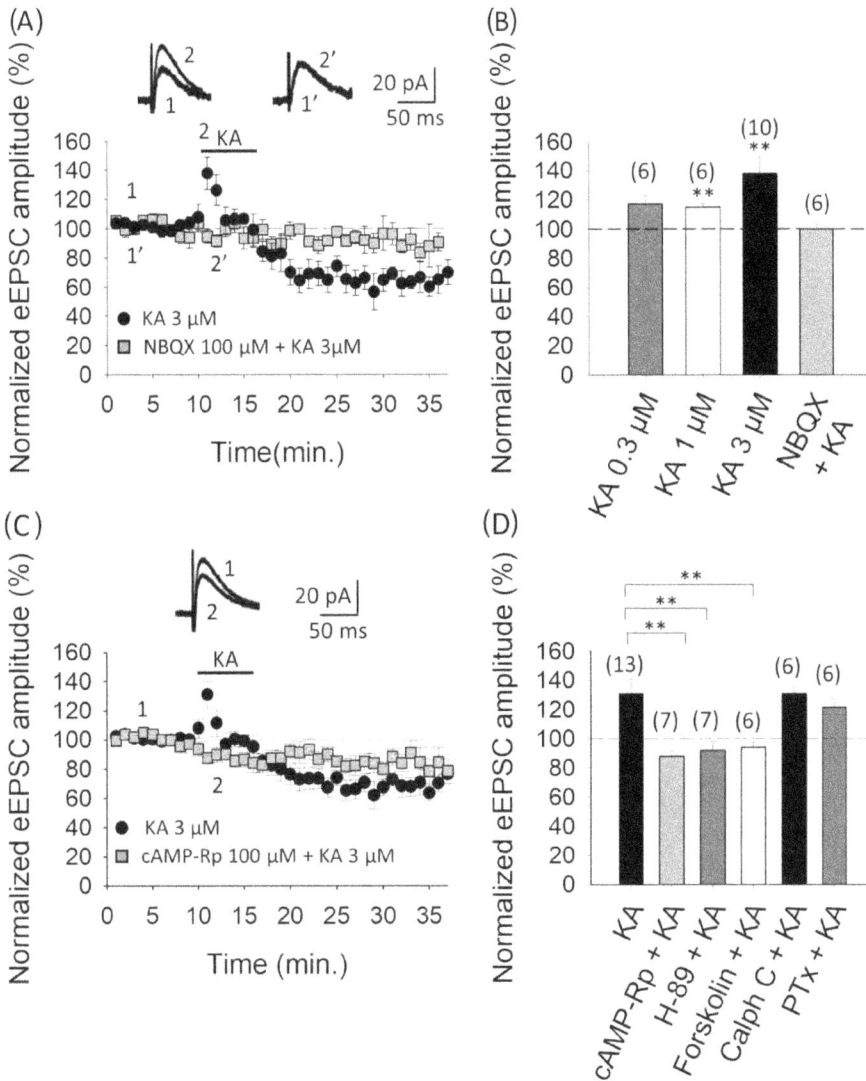

Figure 1.
KAR-mediated facilitation of glutamate release involving activation of adenylyl cyclase (AC) and downstream protein kinase A (PKA) at PF-PuC synapses of the cerebellum. (A) Time course of KA (3 μM) effect on eEPSCs amplitude in the absence (circles) and presence of NBQX (squares). Insets show traces before and after 4 min of KA perfusion in the absence (1, 2) and in the presence of 10 μM NBQX (1', 2'). (B) Quantification of modulation observed in (A) and dose-response curve. (C) Time course of the effect of KA on eEPSC amplitude in cAMP-Rp-treated slices. (D) Inhibition of PKA by cAMP-Rp (100 μM) or H-89 (2 μM), and activation of AC by forskolin (30 μM) prevented the facilitatory action of KA. Inhibition of PKC with calphostin C (1 μM) has no effect on the KA enhancement of the eEPSC amplitude. The facilitatory effect of KA is not affected in slices treated with pertussis toxin. Modified from [64].

was observed as reported for other different brain areas including thalamus, cortex, hippocampus, and amygdala [89–92]. This depression of glutamate release was prevented in the presence of cAMP-RP (which inhibits the activation of PKA), but was not affected by any other experimental modification discussed above with respect to the facilitation of glutamate release. This fact may indicate that the synaptic depression is probably related to an AC/cAMP/PKA signaling pathway (as for facilitation of glutamate release), but without the coupling of Ca^{2+} to the AC. Therefore,

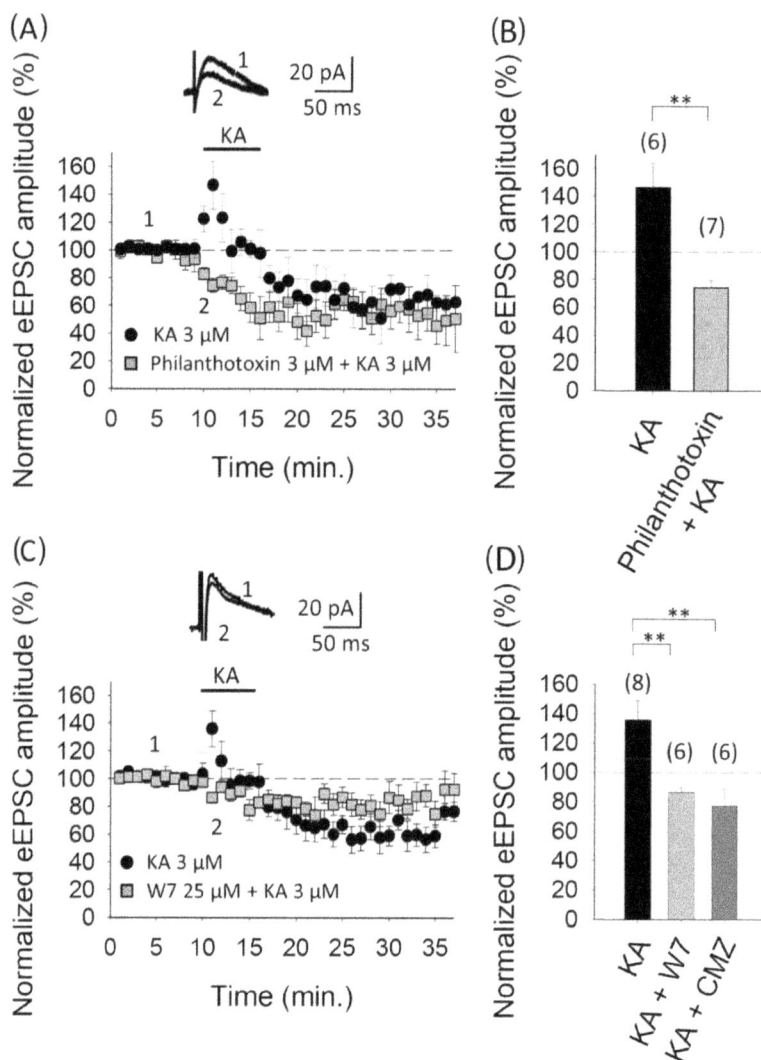

Figure 2.
Facilitation of glutamate release mediated by KAR activation requires an increase of Ca^{2+} in the cytosol and Ca^{2+} calmodulin at cerebellar PF-PuC synapses. (A) Time course of KA (3 μM) effect on eEPSCs amplitude in control condition (circles) and in slices treated with philanthotoxin (squares). (B) Quantification of modulation observed in (A). (C) Time course of KA (3 μM) effect on eEPSCs amplitude in control condition (circles) and in the slices treated with 25 μM W-7 (squares). (D) Quantification of modulation observed in (A). and in the presence of 1 μM CMZ. Modified from [64].

KA receptors have alternative mechanisms for facilitating and depressing glutamate release at PF-Pu synapses (**Figures 1–3**). In previous studies, investigating mossy fiber-CA3 hippocampal synapses [88, 89, 93, 94], as well as the amygdala [37] and cortex [36], a similar mechanism has been observed additionally involving the activation of a G-protein for the depressive effect that may well be also the case for these cerebellar synapses.

Although the presynaptic function of KARs facilitating glutamate release implies an increase in AC/cAMP/PKA signaling induced by the calcium calmodulin complex, KARs appear to be negatively associated with this pathway to carry out synaptic transmission of depression. Previous studies at hippocampal MF-CA3

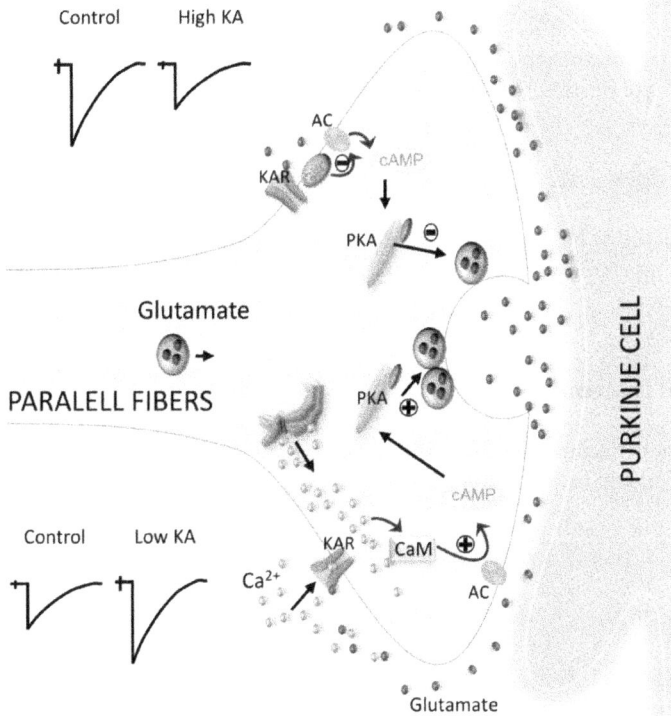

Figure 3.
KAR-mediated modulation of glutamate release in the cerebellum. Actions of KARs depressing or facilitating glutamate release at the PF-PuC synapse. KAR activation by high concentrations of KA (>3 μM) depresses glutamate release at PF-PuC synapses, an effect that involves $G_{i/o}$ protein and the adenylate cyclase/cAMP/ protein kinase A (AC/cAMP/PKA) pathway. KAR activation by low concentrations of kainate (<0.3 μM) only facilitates glutamate release following activation of a Ca^{2+}-calmodulin/AC/cAMP/PKA pathway.

synapses and thalamocortical synapses, as well as at PF-PuC synapses, have reported that the depression of glutamate release mediated by presynaptic KARs occurs through a negative coupling to the AC/cAMP/PKA pathway, being actually evoked by the action of a PTx-sensitive protein G [80, 88, 92]. Despite the hypotheses discussed above, it is also possible that these observed mechanisms reflect the presence of two different types of KARs, a clear objective being to clarify this hypothesis in future studies.

3. Conclusions

Regarding the role and mechanisms of KARs in the modulation of glutamate release in the cerebellum, new and recent data indicate that the KARs effecting facilitation of glutamate release and synaptic transmission show a mandatory dependence on adenylyl cyclase (AC) and cAMP-mediated protein kinase A (PKA) activity. Furthermore, the KAR-mediated facilitation of transmission is contingent on both external Ca^{2+} permeation into the cytosol through KAR and repletion of intracellular Ca^{2+} stores. Finally, a major sensitivity of facilitation to calmodulin inhibition suggests that KARs are coupled through a Ca^{2+}-calmodulin/AC/cAMP/PKA pathway at PF-PuC synapses in the cerebellum. KARs seem to use the inhibition of the AC/cAMP/PKA pathway to mediate a depression of glutamate release at the same synapses, but the activation of the AC does not involve calcium calmodulin and seems to be directly activated by a PTX-sensitive G protein.

Acknowledgements

Work related to kainate receptors in the corresponding author AR-M's laboratory has been supported by Spanish Ministry of Education and Fundación Rodríguez-Pascual grants.

Conflict of interest

The authors declare that the research was conducted in the absence of any commercial or financial relationships that could be construed as a potential conflict of interest.

Author details

Pilar Losada-Ruiz, Rafael Falcón-Moya and Antonio Rodríguez-Moreno*
Department of Physiology, Anatomy and Cell Biology, Pablo de Olavide University, Seville, Spain

*Address all correspondence to: arodmor@upo.es

IntechOpen

© 2019 The Author(s). Licensee IntechOpen. This chapter is distributed under the terms of the Creative Commons Attribution License (http://creativecommons.org/licenses/by/3.0), which permits unrestricted use, distribution, and reproduction in any medium, provided the original work is properly cited. (cc) BY

References

[1] Lerma J, Paternain A, Rodríguez-Moreno A, López-García JC. Molecular physiology of kainate receptors. Physiological Reviews. 2001;**81**:971-998. DOI: 10.1152/physrev.2001.81.3.971

[2] Traynelis SF, Wollmuth LP, McBain CJ, Menniti FS, Vance KM, Ogden KK, et al. Glutamate receptor ion channels: Structure, regulation, and function. Pharmacological Reviews. 2010;**62**: 405-496. DOI: 10.1124/pr.109.002451

[3] Flores G, Negrete-Díaz JV, Carrión M, Andrade-Talavera Y, Bello SA, Sihra TS, et al. Excitatory amino acids in neurological and neurodegenerative disorders. In: Amino Acids in Human Nutrition and Health. Wallingford: CAB International; 2011. pp. 427-453

[4] Niswender CM, Conn PJ. Metabotropic glutamate receptors: Physiology, pharmacology, and disease. Annual Review of Pharmacology and Toxicology. 2010;**50**:295-322. DOI: 10.1146/annurev.pharmtox.011008.145533

[5] Nadler JV, Perry BW, Cotman CW. Intraventricular kainic acid preferentially destroys hippocampal pyramidal cells. Nature. 1978;**271**:676-677. DOI: 10.1038/271676a0

[6] Falcón-Moya R, Sihra TS, Rodríguez-Moreno A. Kainate receptors: Role in epilepsy. Frontiers in Molecular Neuroscience. 2018;**11**:217. DOI: 10.3389/fnmol.2018.00217

[7] Lerma J, Marques JM. Kainate receptors in health and disease. Neuron. 2013;**80**(2):292-311. DOI: 10.1016/j.neuron.2013.09.045

[8] Paternain AV, Rodríguez-Moreno A, Villarroel A, Lerma J. Activation and desensitization properties of native and recombinant kainate receptors. Neuropharmacology. 1998;**37**(10-11):1249-1259

[9] Lee DL, editor. The Biology of the Nematodes. Boca Raton: CRC Press. Taylor and Francis Group; 2010

[10] Li Y, Dharkar P, Han TH, Serpe M, Lee CH, Mayer ML. Novel functional properties of Drosophila CNS glutamate receptors. Neuron. 2016;**92**(5):1036-1048

[11] Somogyi P, Eshhar N, Teichberg VI, Roberts JDB. Subcellular localization of a putative kainate receptor in Bergmann glial cells using a monoclonal antibody in the chick and fish cerebellar cortex. Neuroscience. 1990;**35**(1):9-30

[12] Atoji Y, Sarkar S. Localization of AMPA, kainate, and NMDA receptor mRNAs in the pigeon cerebellum. Journal of Chemical Neuroanatomy. 2019;**98**:71-79

[13] Estabel J, König N, Exbrayat JM. AMPA/kainate receptors permeable to divalent cations in amphibian central nervous system. Life Sciences. 1999;**64**(8):607-616

[14] Huettner JE. Kainate receptors and synaptic transmission. Progress in Neurobiology. 2003;**70**(5):387-407. DOI: 10.1016/S0301-0082(03)00122-9

[15] Jane DE, Lodge D, Collingridge GL. Kainate receptors: Pharmacology, function and therapeutic potential. Neuropharmacology. 2009;**56**(1):90-113. DOI: 10.1016/j.neuropharm.2008.08.023

[16] Paternain AV, Herrera MT, Nieto MA, Lerma J. GluR5 and GluR6 kainate receptor subunits coexist in hippocampal neurons and coassemble to form functional receptors. Journal of Neuroscience. 2000;**20**(1):196-205. DOI: 10.1523/JNEUROSCI.20-01-00196.2000

[17] Rodríguez-Moreno A, Sihra TS. Metabotropic actions of kainate receptors in the CNS. Journal of

Neurochemistry. 2007;**103**(6):2121-2135. DOI: 10.1111/j.1471-4159.2007.04924.x

[18] Rodríguez-Moreno A, Sihra TS. Kainate receptors with a metabotropic modus operandi. Trends in Neurosciences. 2007;**30**(12):630-637. DOI: 10.1016/j.tins.2007.10.001

[19] Sihra TS, Rodríguez-Moreno A. Metabotropic actions of kainate receptors in the control of GABA release. In: Kainate Receptors. Boston, MA: Springer; 2011. pp. 1-10

[20] Rodríguez-Moreno A, Sihra TS. Metabotropic actions of kainate receptors in the control of glutamate release in the hippocampus. In: Kainate Receptors. Boston, MA: Springer; 2011. pp. 39-48

[21] Sihra TS, Rodríguez-Moreno A. Presynaptic kainate receptor-mediated bidirectional modulatory actions: Mechanisms. Neurochemistry International. 2013;**62**(7):982-987. DOI: 10.1016/j.neuint.2013.03.012

[22] Negrete-Díaz JV, Sihra TS, Flores G, Rodríguez-Moreno A. Non-canonical mechanisms of presynaptic kainate receptors controlling glutamate release. Frontiers in Molecular Neuroscience. 2018;**11**:128. DOI: 10.3389/fnmol.2018.00128

[23] Sihra TS, Flores G, Rodríguez-Moreno A. Kainate receptors: Multiple roles in neuronal plasticity. The Neuroscientist. 2014;**20**(1):29-43. DOI: 10.1177/1073858413478196

[24] Rodríguez-Moreno A, Herreras O, Lerma J. Kainate receptors presynaptically downregulate GABAergic inhibition in the rat hippocampus. Neuron. 1997;**19**(4):893-901. DOI: 10.1016/S0896-6273(00)80970-8

[25] Mulle C, Sailer A, Pérez-Otaño I, Dickinson-Anson H, Castillo PE, Bureau I, et al. Altered synaptic physiology and reduced susceptibility to kainite-induced seizures in GluR6-deficient mice. Nature. 1998;**392**:601-605

[26] Smolders I, Bortolotto ZA, Clarke VR, Warre R, Khan GM, O'Neill MJ, et al. Antagonists of GLU(K5)-containing kainate receptors prevent pilocarpine-induced limbic seizures. Nature Neuroscience. 2002;**5**(8):796-804

[27] Fritsch B, Reis J, Gasior M, Kaminski RM, Rogawski MA. Role of GluK1 kainate receptors in seizures, epileptic discharges, and epileptogenesis. The Journal of Neuroscience. 2014;**34**(17):5765-5775. DOI: 10.1523/JNEUROSCI.5307-13.2014

[28] Rodríguez-Moreno A, Lerma J. Kainate receptor modulation of GABA release involves a metabotropic function. Neuron. 1998;**20**(6):1211-1218. DOI: 10.1016/S0896-6273(00)80501-2

[29] Rodríguez-Moreno A, López-García JC, Lerma J. Two populations of kainate receptors with separate signaling mechanisms in hippocampal interneurons. Proceedings of the National Academy of Sciences. 2000;**97**(3):1293-1298. DOI: 10.1073/pnas.97.3.1293

[30] Artinian J, Peret A, Marti G, Epsztein J, Crépel V. Synaptic kainate receptors in interplay with INaP shift the sparse firing of dentate granule cells to a sustained rhythmic mode in temporal lobe epilepsy. The Journal of Neuroscience. 2011;**31**(30):10811-10818. DOI: 10.1523/JNEUROSCI.0388-11.2011

[31] Artinian J, Peret A, Mircheva Y, Marti G, Crépel V. Impaired neuronal operation through aberrant intrinsic plasticity in epilepsy. Annals of Neurology. 2015;**77**(4):592-606. DOI: 10.1002/ana.24348

[32] Peret A, Christie LA, Ouedraogo DW, Gorlewicz A, Epsztein J, Mulle C, et al. Contribution of aberrant GluK2-containing kainate receptors to chronic seizures in temporal lobe epilepsy. Cell Reports. 2014;**8**(2):347-354. DOI: 10.1016/j.celrep.2014.06.032

[33] Crépel V, Mulle C. Physiopathology of kainate receptors in epilepsy. Current Opinion in Pharmacology. 2015;**20**:83-88. DOI: 10.1016/j.coph.2014.11.012

[34] Sander T, Hildmann T, Kretz R, Fürst R, Sailer U, Bauer G, et al. Allelic association of juvenile absence epilepsy with a GluR5 kainate receptor gene (GRIK1) polymorphism. American Journal of Medical Genetics. 1997;**74**:416-421

[35] Li JM, Zeng YJ, Peng F, Li L, Yang TH, Hong Z, et al. Aberrant glutamate receptor 5 expression in temporal lobe epilepsy lesions. Brain Research. 2010;**1311**:166-174

[36] Swanson GT. Targeting AMPA and kainate receptors in neurological disease: Therapies on the horizon? Neuropsychopharmacology. 2009;**34**:249-250

[37] Sanchez-Gomez MV, Matute C. AMPA and kainate receptors each mediate excitotoxicity in oligodendroglial cultures. Neurobiology of Disease. 1999;**6**:475-485. DOI: 10.1006/nbdi.1999.0264

[38] Matute C. Characteristics of acute and chronic kainate excitotoxic damage to the optic nerve. Proceedings of the National Academy of Sciences of the United States of America. 1998;**95**:10229-10234. DOI: 10.1073/pnas.95.17.10229

[39] Tekkok SB, Goldberg MP. AMPA/kainate receptor activation mediates hypoxic oligodendrocyte death and axonal injury in cerebral white matter. The Journal of Neuroscience.

2001;**21**:4237-4248. DOI: 10.1523/JNEUROSCI.21-12-04237.2001

[40] Xu J, Liu Y, Zhang GY. Neuroprotection of GluR5-containing kainate receptor activation again ischemic brain injury through decreasing tyrosine phosphorylation of N-methyl-D-aspartate reeptors mediated by SRC kinase. The Journal of Biological Chemistry. 2008;**283**:29355-29366

[41] O'Neill MJ, Bogaert L, Hicks CA, Bond A, Ward MA, Ebinger G, et al. LY377770, a novel iGlu5 kainate receptor antagonist with neuroprotective effects in global and focal cerebral ischaemia. Neuropharmacology. 2000;**39**:1575-1588. DOI: 10.1016/S0028-3908(99)00250-6

[42] Aronica E, Dickson DW, Kress Y, Morrison JH, Zukin RS. Non-plaque dystrophic dendrites in Alzheimer hippocampus: A new pathological structure revealed by glutamate receptor immunocytochemistry. Neuroscience. 1998;**82**:979-991. DOI: 10.1016/S0306-4522(97)00260-1

[43] Luquim MR, Saldise L, Guillén J, et al. Does increased excitatory drive from the subthalamic nucleus contribute to dopaminergic neuronal death in Parkinson's disease? Experimental Neurology. 2006;**201**:407-415

[44] Carson KM, Andresen JM, Orr HT. Emerging pathogenic pathways in the spinocerebellar ataxias. Current Opinion in Genetics and Development. 2009;**19**:247-253

[45] Wagster MV, Hedreen JC, Peyser CE, Folstein SE, Ross CA. Selective loss of [3H] kainic acid and [3H] AMPA binding in layer VI of frontal cortex in Huntington's disease. Experimental Neurology. 1994;**127**:70-75. DOI: 10.1006/exnr.1994.1081

[46] Rubinsztein DC, Leggo J, Chiano M, Dodge A, Norbury G, Rosser E, et al.

Genotypes at the GluR6 kainate receptor locus are associated with variation in the age of onset of Huntington disease. Proceedings of the National Academy of Sciences of the United States of America. 1997;**94**:3872-3876. DOI: 10.1073/pnas.94.8.3872

[47] MacDonald ME, Vonsattel JP, Shrinidhi J, Couropmitree NN, Cupples LA, Bird ED, et al. Evidence for the GluR6 gene associated with younger onset age of Huntington's disease. Neurology. 1999;**53**:1330-1332. DOI: 10.1212/WNL.53.6.1330

[48] Garey LJ, Von Bussmann KA, Hirsch SR. Decreasednumerical density of kainate receptor-positive neurons in the orbitofrontal cortex of chronic schizophrenics. Experimental Brain Research. 2006;**173**:234-242. DOI: 10.1007/s00221-006-0396-8

[49] Begni S, Popoli M, Moraschi S, Bignotti S, Tura GB, Gennarelli M. Association between the ionotropic glutamate receptor kainate 3 (GRIK3) ser310ala polymorphism and schizophrenia. Molecular Psychiatry. 2002;**7**:416-418. DOI: 10.1038/sj.mp.4000987

[50] Schiffer HH, Heinemann SF. Association of the human kainate receptor GluR7 gene (GRIK3) with recurrent major depressive disorder. American Journal of Medical Genetics. Part B, Neuropsychiatric Genetics. 2007;**144**:20-26. DOI: 10.1002/ajmg.b.30374

[51] Pickard BS, Malloy MP, Christoforou A, et al. Cytogenetic and genetic evidence supports a role for the kainate-type glutamate receptor gene, GRIK4, in schizophrenia and bipolar disorder. Molecular Psychiatry. 2006;**11**:847-857. DOI: 10.1038/sj.mp.4001867

[52] Wilson GM, Flibotte S, Chopra V, Melnyk BL, Honer WG, Holt RA. DNA copy number analysis in bipolar disorder and schizophrenia reveals aberrations in genes involved in glutamate signaling. Human Molecular Genetics. 2006;**15**:743-749. DOI: 10.1093/hmg/ddi489

[53] Motazacker MM, Rost BR, Hucho T, Garshasbi M, Kahrizi K, Ullmann R, et al. A defect in the ionotropic glutamate receptor 6 gene (GRIK2) is associated with autosomal recessive mental retardation. American Journal of Human Genetics. 2007;**81**:792-798. DOI: 10.1086/521275

[54] Jamain S, Betancur C, Mol Quach H, Philippe A, Fellous M, Giros B, et al. Linkage and association of the glutamate receptor 6 gene with autism. Molecular Psychiatry. 2002;**7**:302-310. DOI: 10.1038/sj.mp.4000979

[55] Bowie D. Ionotropic glutamate receptors & CNS disorders. CNS & Neurological Disorders Drug Targets. 2008;**7**:129-143

[56] Matute C. Therapeutic potential of kainate receptors. CNS Neuroscience and Therapeutics. 2011;**17**(6):661-669. DOI: 10.1111/j.1755-5949.2010.00204.x

[57] Pemberton KE, Belcher SM, Ripellino JA, Howe JR. High-affinity kainate-type ion channels in rat cerebellar granule cells. The Journal of Physiology. 1998;**510**(2):401-420. DOI: 10.1111/j.1469-7793.1998.401bk.x

[58] Smith TC, Wang LY, Howe JR. Distinct kainate receptor phenotypes in immature and mature mouse cerebellar granule cells. The Journal of Physiology. 1999;**517**(1):51-58. DOI: 10.1111/j.1469-7793.1999.0051z.x

[59] Spiliopoulos K, Fragioudaki K, Giompres P, Kouvelas E, Mitsacos A. Expression of GluR6 kainate receptor subunit in granular layer of weaver mouse cerebellum. Journal of Neural Transmission. 2009;**116**(4):417-422. DOI: 10.1007/s00702-009-0199-8

[60] Tyrrell T, Willshaw D. Cerebellar cortex: Its simulation and the relevance of Marr's theory. Philosophical Transactions of the Royal Society of London. Series B: Biological Sciences. 1992;**336**(1277):239-257. DOI: 10.1098/rstb.1992.0059

[61] Wadiche JI, Jahr CE. Multivesicular release at climbing fiber-Purkinje cell synapses. Neuron. 2001;**32**(2):301-313. DOI: 10.1016/S0896-6273(01)00488-3

[62] Crépel F. Role of presynaptic kainate receptors at parallel-fiber-purkinje cell synapses in induction of cerebellar LTD: Interplay with climbing fiber input. Journal of Neurophysiology. 2009;**102**:965-973

[63] Rodríguez-Moreno A, Paulsen O. Spike timing-dependent long-term depression requires presynaptic NMDA receptors. Nature Neuroscience. 2008;**11**:744-745

[64] Banerjee A, Meredith RM, Rodríguez-Moreno A, Mierau SB, Auberson YP, Paulsen O. Double dissociation of spike timing-dependent potentiation and depression by subunit-preferring NMDA receptors antagonists in mouse barrel cortex. Cerebral Cortex. 2009;**19**:2959-2969

[65] Rodríguez-Moreno A, Banerjee A, Paulsen O. Presynaptic NMDA receptors and spike timing-dependent depression at cortical synapses. Frontiers in Synaptic Neuroscience. 2010;**2**:18. DOI: 10.3389/fnsyn.2010.00018

[66] Rodríguez-Moreno A, Kohl MM, Reeve J, Eaton TR, Collins HA, Anderson HL, et al. Presynaptic induction and expression of timing-dependent long-term depression demonstrated by compartment specific photorelease of a use-dependent NMDA antagonist. The Journal of Neuroscience. 2011;**31**:8564-8569

[67] Buchanan KA, Blackman AV, Moreau AW, Elgar D, Costa RP, Lalanne

T, et al. Target-specific expression of presynaptic NMDA receptors in neocortical microcircuits. Neuron. 2012;**75**:451-466

[68] Rodríguez-Moreno A, González-Rueda A, Banerjee A, Upton ML, Craig M, Paulsen O. Presynaptic self-depression at developing neocortical synapses. Neuron. 2013;**77**:35-42

[69] Banerjee A, González-Rueda A, Sampaio-Baptista C, Paulse O, Rodríguez-Moreno A. Distinct mechanisms of spike timing-dependent LTD at vertical and horizontal inputs onto L2/3 pyramidal neurons in mouse barrel cortex. Physiological Reports. 2014;**2**(3):1-11. DOI: 10.1002/phy2.271

[70] Komuro H, Rakic P. Modulation of neuronal migration by NMDA receptors. Science. 1993;**260**(5104):95-97. DOI: 10.1126/science.8096653

[71] Rabacchi S, Bailly Y, Delhaye-Bouchaud N, Mariani J. Involvement of the N-methyl D-aspartate (NMDA) receptor in synapse elimination during cerebellar development. Science. 1992;**256**(5065):1823-1825. DOI: 10.1126/science.1352066

[72] Maiti A, Salles KS, Grassi S, Abood LG. Behavior and receptor changes after kainate lesioning of nodular cerebellum. Pharmacology Biochemistry and Behavior. 1986;**25**(3):589-594. DOI: 10.1016/0091-3057(86)90146-2

[73] de Vera N, Camón L, Martínez E. Cerebral distribution of polyamines in kainic acid-induced models of status epilepticus and ataxia in rats. Overproduction of putrescine and histological damage. European Neuropsychopharmacology. 2002;**12**(5):397-405. DOI: 10.1016/S0924-977X(02)00050-0

[74] Yamaguchi T, Hayashi K, Murakami H, Maruyama S, Yamaguchi M. Distribution and characterization of

the glutamate receptors in the CNS of ataxic mutant mouse. Neurochemical Research. 1984;**9**(4):497-505. DOI: 10.1007/BF00964376

[75] Andoh T, Kishi H, Motoki K, Nakanishi K, Kuraishi Y, Muraguchi A. Protective effect of IL-18 on kainate- and IL-1 β-induced cerebellar ataxia in mice. Journal of Immunology. 2008;**180**:2322-2328. DOI: 10.4049/jimmunol.180.4.2322

[76] Harrison PJ, Barton AJ, Najlerahim A, Pearson RC. Distribution of a kainate/AMPA receptor mRNA in normal and Alzheimer brain. Neuroreport. 1990;**1**(2):149-152

[77] Bullock WM, Cardon K, Bustillo J, Roberts RC, Perrone-Bizzozero NI. Altered expression of genes involved in GABAergic transmission and neuromodulation of granule cell activity in the cerebellum of schizophrenia patients. American Journal of Psychiatry. 2008;**165**(12):1594-1603. DOI: 10.1176/appi.ajp.2008.07121845

[78] Korf J, Postema F. Regional calcium accumulation and cation shifts in rat brain by kainate. Journal of Neurochemistry. 1984;**43**(4):1052-1060. DOI: 10.1111/j.1471-4159.1984.tb12843.x

[79] Savidge JR, Bleakman D, Bristow DR. Identification of kainate receptor-mediated intracellular calcium increases in cultured rat cerebellar granule cells. Journal of Neurochemistry. 1997;**69**(4):1763-1766. DOI: 10.1046/j.1471-4159.1997.69041763.x

[80] Falcón-Moya R, Losada-Ruiz P, Sihra TS, Rodríguez-Moreno A. Cerebellar Kainate receptor-mediated facilitation of glutamate release requires Ca^{2+}−calmodulin and PKA. Frontiers in Molecular Neuroscience. 2018;**11**:1-10. DOI: 10.3389/fnmol.2018.00195

[81] Bahn S, Volk B, Wisden W. Kainate receptor gene expression in the developing rat brain. Journal of Neuroscience. 1994;**14**(9):5525-5547. DOI: 10.1523/JNEUROSCI.14-09-05525.1994

[82] Bettler B, Boulter J, Hermans-Borgmeyer I, O'Shea-Greenfield A, Deneris ES, Moll C, et al. Cloning of a novel glutamate receptor subunit, GluR5: Expression in the nervous system during development. Neuron. 1990;**5**(5):583-595. DOI: 10.1016/0896-6273(90)90213-y

[83] Herb A, Burnashev N, Werner P, Sakmann B, Wisden W, Seeburg PH. The KA-2 subunit of excitatory amino acid receptors shows widespread expression in brain and forms ion channels with distantly related subunits. Neuron. 1992;**8**(4):775-785. DOI: 10.1016/0896-6273(92)90098-x

[84] Petralia RS, Wang YX, Wenthold RJ. Histological and ultrastructural localization of the kainate receptor subunits, KA2 and GluR6/7, in the rat nervous system using selective antipeptide antibodies. Journal of Comparative Neurology. 1994;**349**(1):85-110. DOI: 10.1002/cne.903490107

[85] Swanson GT, Feldmeyer D, Kaneda M, Cull-Candy SG. Effect of RNA editing and subunit co-assembly single-channel properties of recombinant kainate receptors. Journal of Physiology. 1996;**492**:129-142

[86] Delaney AJ, Jahr CE. Kainate receptors differentially regulate release at two parallel fiber synapses. Neuron. 2002;**36**(3):475-482. DOI: 10.1016/s08966273(02)01008-5

[87] Rodríguez-Moreno A, Sihra TS. Presynaptic kainate receptor facilitation of glutamate release involves protein kinase A in the rat hippocampus. Journal of Physiology. 2004;**557**(3):733-745. DOI: 10.1113/jphysiol.2004.065029

[88] Negrete-Díaz JV, Sihra TS, Delgado-García JM, Rodríguez-Moreno A. Kainate receptor–mediated inhibition of glutamate release involves protein kinase A in the mouse hippocampus. Journal of Neurophysiology. 2006;**96**(4):1829-1837. DOI: 10.1152/jn.00280.2006

[89] Andrade-Talavera Y, Duque-Feria P, Negrete-Díaz JV, Sihra TS, Flores G, Rodríguez-Moreno A. Presynaptic kainate receptor-mediated facilitation of glutamate release involves Ca^{2+}-calmodulin at mossy fiber-CA3 synapses. Journal of Neurochemistry. 2012;**122**(5):891-899. DOI: 10.1111/j.1471-4159.2012.07844.x

[90] Rodríguez-Moreno A, Sihra TS. Presynaptic kainate receptor-mediated facilitation of glutamate release involves Ca^{2+}–calmodulin and PKA in cerebrocortical synaptosomes. FEBS Letters. 2013;**587**(6):788-792. DOI: 10.1016/j.febslet.2013.01.071

[91] Negrete-Díaz JV, Duque-Feria P, Andrade-Talavera Y, Carrión M, Flores G, Rodríguez-Moreno A. Kainate receptor-mediated depression of glutamatergic transmission involving protein kinase A in the lateral amygdala. Journal of Neurochemistry. 2012;**121**(1):36-43. DOI: 10.1111/j.1471-4159.2012.07665.x

[92] Andrade-Talavera Y, Duque-Feria P, Sihra TS, Rodríguez-Moreno A. Pre-synaptic kainate receptor-mediated facilitation of glutamate release involves PKA and Ca^{2+}-calmodulin at thalamocortical synapses. Journal of Neurochemistry. 2013;**126**(5):565-578. DOI: 10.1016/j.febslet.2013.01.071

[93] Negrete-Díaz JV, Sihra TS, Delgado-García JM, Rodríguez-Moreno A. Kainate receptor-mediated presynaptic inhibition converges with presynaptic inhibition mediated by Group II mGluRs and long-term depression at the hippocampal mossy fiber-CA3 synapse. Journal of Neural Transmission. 2007;**114**(11):1425-1431. DOI: 10.1007/s00702-007-0750-4

[94] Lyon L, Borel M, Carrión M, Kew JN, Corti C, Harrison PJ, et al. Hippocampal mossy fiber long-term depression in Grm2/3 double knockout mice. Synapse. 2011;**65**(9):945-954. DOI: 10.1002/syn.20923

Chapter 3

Homeostatic Plasticity and Therapeutic Approaches in Neurodegeneration

Sagrario Martin-Aragon, Paloma Bermejo-Bescós,
Pilar González and Juana Benedí

Abstract

The synapses transmit signals between neurons in an ever-changing fashion. Changes of synaptic transmission arise from numerous mechanisms known as synaptic plasticity. The importance and complexity of the synapse has fueled research into the molecular mechanisms underlying synaptogenesis, synaptic transmission, and plasticity. Particularly, homeostatic plasticity refers to the local changes in synaptic activation to generate local synaptic adaptations and network-wide changes in activity to generate adjustments between excitation and inhibition. This review chapter will focus on synaptic phenomena and mechanisms that are likely to contribute to network homeostasis. In addition, it will be discussed a putative modulation of the signaling mechanisms serving a homeostatic function as a viable therapeutic approach for disease modification in neurological and neurodegenerative disorders. To sum up, the main role of the following players in homeostatic plasticity will be analyzed, based on what a growing body of evidence has suggested recently: BDNF-mediated TrkB system activation; adenosine modulation system; nitric oxide/soluble GC/cGMP signaling; astrocyte involvement—astroglial CB1 receptors; the microtubule-associated neuronal protein Tau; the signaling pathway of the Wnt protein family; extracellular vesicles in the intercellular communication; and estrogen involvement in non-reproductive functions.

Keywords: adenosine, astrocytes, BDNF, estrogens, extracellular vesicles, neurodegeneration, nitric oxide, synaptic plasticity, Tau, TrkB system, Wnt proteins

1. Introduction

The neurotransmission may be defined as the set of biochemical and physiochemical signals which establishes neuronal communication. Changes of synaptic transmission arise from numerous mechanisms known as synaptic plasticity. Synaptic plasticity is crucial for regulating synaptic transmission or electrical signal transduction to neuronal networks, for sharing essential information among neurons and for maintaining homeostasis in the body.

Synaptic plasticity in the mature nervous system includes structural and morphological modifications constituting the cellular response to the changes in neuronal activity that are thought to be responsible for learning and memory [1].

The individual synaptic connections are constantly removed or recreated depending on the neuronal environment. This plasticity is highly regulated by signals from other cells of the nervous system, mainly the astrocytes whose function is the maintenance of the neurons in a determined position [2]. This modeling ability is achieved by genetic, molecular, and cellular mechanisms that influence synaptic connections and neuronal circuits.

Various neurotransmitter receptors are functionally associated with protein kinases and other G-proteins that modulate cascades of molecules which in turn maintain essential cellular functions [3]. Modifications of the MAPK- and cAMP-related signaling pathways may affect intracellular Ca^{2+} levels, neurotransmitter receptors, transcription factors, and the cross-link between signaling pathways, among other biological functions which are essential for neuroplasticity [4].

At the structural level, synaptic plasticity entails incorporation or disassociation of α-amino-3-hydroxy-5-methyl-isoxazole-4-propionic acid (AMPA) receptors from the postsynaptic membrane and the growth or constriction of the dendritic spines where most excitatory synapses are placed [5]. At the functional level, synaptic plasticity is considered as the long-term potentiation (LTP) or long-term depression (LTD) of synaptic strength, with modifications in conductance through AMPA receptors in the postsynaptic membrane. During the term of plasticity, N-methyl-D-aspartate (NMDA) receptor activation leads to Ca^{2+} ions passage through the postsynaptic membrane to trigger intracellular signaling cascades. These events set off gene transcription, trafficking of AMPA receptor via action dynamics, cytoskeleton reorganization, and enlargement or removal of dendritic spines. The integrity of the synaptic structure, trafficking of AMPA receptor, and dendritic spine dynamics are all crucial for generating lasting synaptic plasticity modifications [5].

The AMPA receptors and NMDA receptors are the ones which synergize at postsynaptic terminals to facilitate different forms of synaptic plasticity. Constant activation of AMPA receptors by a series of impulses arriving at presynaptic terminals leads to depolarization of the presynaptic membrane, which removes the Mg^{2+} ions that are obstructed at NMDA receptors [6]. Thereon, the simultaneous excitation of pre- and postsynaptic neurons speeds up the gating of NMDA channels and reinforces the synapse. This feature is crucial in NMDA channels for being specifically associated with synaptic plasticity and its high permeability to Ca^{2+} ions. Therefore, the second messenger Ca^{2+} modulates a set of signaling pathways and the responses that collectively lead to synaptic modification [6].

Furthermore, local changes in synaptic activation to generate local synaptic adaptations and network-wide changes in activity result in adjustments between excitation and inhibition. These mechanisms are likely to contribute to network homeostasis. Therefore, this review chapter will focus on synaptic phenomena involved in homeostatic plasticity. In addition, it will be discussed a putative modulation of the signaling mechanisms serving a homeostatic function as a viable therapeutic approach for disease modification in neurological and neurodegenerative disorders.

2. BDNF-mediated TrkB system activation

Synaptic plasticity at the molecular level can be driven by increased expression of plasticity-related genes, such as brain-derived neurotrophic factor (BDNF), calcium/calmodulin kinase II (CaMKII), and cAMP response element binding (CREB) protein, as well as by an augmented expression of both AMPA and NMDA receptors on surface [7].

The escalation of the synapse is a mode of homeostatic plasticity in which a prolonged enhancement in neuronal activity leads to a compensatory decline in excitatory transmission that is often mediated by a drop in levels of the synaptic AMPA receptors. The blockage of sustained activity results in the opposite effect, that is, an enhancement in excitatory transmission that is often mediated by an augmentation in levels of the synaptic AMPA receptors [8]. The neurotrophin BDNF and its signaling partners are the main regulators of synaptic plasticity. BDNF may serve as a real mediator rather than simply a modulator of synaptic plasticity and synaptic communication. As BDNF is synthesized and released in an activity-dependent manner [9], BDNF levels could serve as signals for changes in neuronal activity and thereby mediate synaptic scaling. BDNF and neurotransmitter signaling cascades can work together in close temporal association to induce immediate and guided effects on synaptic plasticity. What is more, specifically interfering with BDNF-related signaling is a crucial strategy for neuronal and functionally restorative treatments for neurological and psychiatric disorders [10].

The main functions of BDNF are mediated by its interaction with the tropomyosin-related kinase B (TrkB) receptor [11] whose intracellular signaling cascade activation can affect synaptic transmission and synaptic contact formation [12]. TrkB receptors are typically localized within vesicles inside the cell and translocate to the plasma membrane through neuronal activity [13]. The early effects of BDNF are a result of the modification (e.g., protein phosphorylation) of components that are already present at the synapse, while the long-term effects originate from the modification of translational activity at the synapse and changes in transcription. Stimulation of high-frequency inducing LTP leads to enhancement of BDNF production [14]. Furthermore, BDNF increases neurotransmitter release and promotes synaptic transmission and LTP [15]. Thus, it is assumable that the effects exerted by BDNF on synaptic plasticity are TrkB mediated.

A recent study has investigated the features of neural network formation and functions in primary hippocampal cultures in the context of chronic BDNF application and TrkB receptor blockage [16]. It has been demonstrated that the blockage of TrkB receptors affected the structures of synapses and even mitochondria, which were not regarded as capable of participating in synaptic modulation for a long period. Nevertheless, it has been shown that TrkB-mediated signaling can affect both the ultrastructural and functional parameters of brain mitochondria, even in normal oxygen and nutrient supply conditions. Chronic TrkB receptor blockade leads to destructive ultrastructural changes in mitochondria, whereas the functional activity of organelles remains intact apparently. Long-term application of BDNF enhances the enzymatic activity of mitochondria, though this modification is not related to changes in ultrastructure of organelles. These findings might demonstrate that TrkB-mediated mitochondrial regulation is associated with functional changes of the enzymatic apparatus of the respiratory chain but not with structural reshaping of organelles. Chronic BDNF application increased the basal oxygen consumption rate via activating respiratory chain complex II [17]. Under oxygen stress conditions, BDNF increases the adaptive potential by impacting the functional parameters of the mitochondrial apparatus. Further research should address whether the TrkB-mediated pathway for influencing mitochondria is generalized (i.e., carried out through nuclear genes) or directed toward an isolated organelle.

A genetically determined high level of BDNF can provide significant adaptive potential to the nervous system, and its neuroprotective effects are induced via the TrkB receptor system [18]. To date, it has been found that BDNF-mediated TrkB system activation accounts for the formation of more complex functionally active neural networks with a great level of efficiency in synaptic transmission. Thus, the TrkB signaling system can be involved in higher cognitive functions.

Recent progress into the etiology of neurological and metabolic diseases has been made with genome-wide association studies. BDNF/TrkB signaling contribution to synaptic development and plasticity, neurite outgrowth, and dendritic spine formation is a possible anatomical correlate of hyperconnectivity in autism-spectrum disorder (ASD) [19] or of hypoconnectivity in monogenic obesity [20].

Growing evidence suggests that BDNF upregulation plays a key role in the increased trophic effects in ASD. Studies on functional image have shown that, in most young ASD patients, cortical regions appear hyperlinked, and cortical thickness and brain size are enhanced [19]. These findings indicate that developing ASD brains may occur in a modified neurotrophic environment as some ASD patients and animal models have shown enhanced levels of BDNF.

Besides that, genome association studies now reveal different candidate obesity genes, most of which are strongly expressed or known to act in the CNS, highlighting the role of the brain in propensity to obesity. In this regard, BDNF is involved in energy metabolism and eating behavior as partial BDNF deficiencies in mouse models cause hyperphagia and obesity. The first case described by disruption of the BDNF gene (11p13) in humans was that of an 8-year-old obese girl, who presented an abnormality in chromosome 11 that altered the BDNF gene in one of the chromosomal breakpoints [21]. This patient with severe hyperphagia and obesity also presented a complex neurobehavioral phenotype, including impaired cognitive function and memory and a distinctive hyperactive behavior.

3. Adenosine modulation system

Adenosine is a ubiquitous molecule that is directly involved in the key processes sustaining cellular viability and adaptability, this is it, the energy charge, redox control, DNA and RNA, and epigenetic control. The role of adenosine in the brain is of great interest since the adenosine receptors are far more abundant in the brain than in any other organ or cell type in mammals [22]. Though there are four plasma membrane metabotropic receptors such as adenosine A1, A2A, A2B, and A3 receptors [23], A1 and A2A receptors are the responsible ones for the effects of adenosine in the brain. A1 receptors (A1R) are the most abundant and widely distributed, while A2A receptors (A2AR) are more abundant in the basal ganglia and in synapses throughout the rest of the brain. Both A1R and A2AR are mostly located in synapses, particularly in glutamatergic synapses, although both receptors are also present in other synapses [24].

Adenosine acts on A1R at a pre-synaptical level decreasing calcium influx and glutamate release, at a post-synaptical level decreasing the activation of ionotropic glutamate receptors and of voltage-sensitive calcium channels as well as hyperpolarizing dendrites through a control of potassium channels. The ability of A1R to control high-frequency-induced synaptic plasticity contrasts with that of A2AR. Thus, A2AR are capable of enhancing the evoked release of glutamate in different brain areas and the function of ionotropic glutamate receptors [25]. Besides, A2AR behave as fine-tuners of other neuromodulation systems, since A2AR activation is a requirement for the synaptic effects of growth factors or neuropeptides. What is more, A2AR activation diminishes the efficiency of pre-synaptic inhibitory systems. Thus, A2AR commute pre-synaptic modulation from inhibitory to facilitatory. Another significant feature of A2AR is that they have also been found in astrocytes and microglia cells, controlling Na^+/K^+-ATPase, the uptake of glutamate, the production of pro-inflammatory cytokines, and the effects potentially contributing to the selective A2AR-mediated control of synaptic plasticity [26].

Different sources of extracellular adenosine activate each of these adenosine receptors in order to control synaptic transmission by A1R and synaptic plasticity by A2AR [27]. The predominant role of adenosine under basal conditions, in excitatory synapses, is an A1R-mediated inhibition of synaptic transmission. Then, an endogenous A1R-mediated inhibitory tonus takes place under most experimental conditions. In contrast, A2AR are only recruited upon higher frequencies of nerve stimulation triggering plastic changes of synaptic efficiency (LTP) [28]. This selectivity is consequence of the adenosine formed by synaptic ecto-nucleotidases upon release of ATP from nerve terminals; high-frequency stimulations are needed to trigger an excessive release of ATP [29] that significantly results in the production of extracellular adenosine near A2AR. These A2AR then enhance the release of glutamate and the activation of NMDA receptors, effectively reinforcing the implementation of LTP [30].

Furthermore, the particular activation of A2AR upon higher frequencies of nerve stimulation favors the solution of the increased feedback inhibitory synaptic mechanisms with increasing frequencies of synaptic recruitment. The higher the stimulation frequency, the greater the extracellular levels of adenosine and of cannabinoids since supramaximal activation of pre-synaptic A1R or of cannabinoid CB1R can block synaptic transmission. The neuromodulator adenosine, by operating high affinity adenosine receptors, restrains transmission via A1 receptor (A1R) or CB1R [31].

In spite of the selective involvement of A2AR that allows simultaneously mitigating pre-synaptic inhibition and strengthening synaptic facilitation at the single synapse level, A1R and A2AR actually collaborate to encode the relevance of information at the level of brain circuits. The implementation of a potentiated transmission in a given synapse will elicit in parallel a process of hetero-synaptic depression involving synaptic strengthening of A1R function in surrounding synapses (with respect to this potentiated synapse). The increased recruitment of a synapse set off the activation of the astrocytic syncytium. Within the domain covered by this syncytium, there will be a greater astrocytic (i.e. non-synaptic) release of ATP [32], which will be degraded by ecto-nucleotidases degrading ATP into adenosine, which is channeled into A1R, further depressing the activity of neighboring synapses (where A2AR are not engaged).

In conclusion, a predominant role of neuronal A2AR in the control of neuronal damage is supported by several studies [33]. Dysfunction and damage of synapses may be triggered by the A2AR that are located synaptically. This synapse impairment is regarded as one of the earliest alterations found in different neurodegenerative disorders ranging from Alzheimer's disease (AD) to depression. Experimentally, it has been shown that blockade of A2AR prevents memory damage in AD models. Therefore, the question arises whether A2AR antagonists might have a therapeutic potential. To give some answer, a triple transgenic AD model (3×-Tg-AD) has been used with a defined onset of memory dysfunction occurring at the age of 4 months. After the onset of memory deficits in 3×-Tg-AD mice, a treatment of 3 weeks with a selective A2AR antagonist has shown to normalize the up-regulation of hippocampal A2AR, restore hippocampal-dependent reference memory, and decrease hippocampal synaptic plasticity and global and glutamatergic synaptic markers as well. These findings may point to a therapeutic-like ability of A2AR antagonists to recover synaptic and memory dysfunction that occur in early AD [34]. It may be assumed a role for A2AR in the early steps of neurodegeneration, whereby the up-regulation of A2AR that occurs at the beginning in synapses upon noxious brain insults [27] would set off an aberrant overenforcement of synaptic plasticity that would interrupt synaptic function and favor the likelihood of excitotoxic destruction of the synapse. A2AR would facilitate synaptic plasticity under physiological conditions, while their up-regulation would lead to a synaptic toxicity that occurs early during the course of neuropsychiatric illnesses. Moreover, the up-regulation and role of A2AR in the astrocyte and microglial control suggest an involvement of A2AR in brain damage, which might also include the control of blood flow and endothelial permeability by these receptors. This entails that multiple cellular sites of action of A2AR would participate in the ongoing process engaged in neurodegeneration [33].

4. Nitric oxide/soluble GC/cGMP signaling in synaptic plasticity

Nitric oxide (NO) plays roles in maintaining synaptic plasticity and in helping to restore plasticity in the neuronal architecture in the CNS. NO is regarded as a chemical transmitter which has essential functions in the mammalian central as well as peripheral nervous system [35]. NO is the second mediator that can activate NMDA receptors. NMDA receptor activation persistently enhances the activity of neuronal nitric oxide synthase (nNOS) in the neuronal cytoplasm. It then catalyzes the generation of endogenous NO from L-arginine followed by the enhanced release of NO from neurons. Activation of these receptors by glutamate stimulates the calcium influx into cells and the generation of NO by NOS, which rapidly stimulates guanylate cyclase and increases cGMP synthesis [36]. Other glutamate receptors, such as AMPA, can also produce NO; this pathway modulates the release of glutamate and dopamine. Nevertheless, AMPA receptor trafficking, expression, and S-nitrosylation activity are maintained by NO. Specifically, the N-ethylmaleimide-sensitive factor (NSF, an ATPase) is high in neurons which binds with GluR2 and the NSF-GluR2 interaction has shown to be important to maintain AMPA-mediated transmission at the synapse [37]. Physiologically, synaptic NSF is S-nitrosylated by NO from neuronal source in the mouse brain. Activation of NMDA receptors increases the NSF-GluR2 interaction, as well as the surface insertion of GluR2. NMDA receptors stimulate NO generation, which enhances NSF S-nitrosylation, stimulates its association with GluR2, and increases the surface expression of GluR2-containing AMPA receptors [38].

Additionally, NO is associated with the storage, uptake, and release of mediators, such as acetylcholine, noradrenaline, GABA, taurine, and a glycine. NO can stimulate its own extrasynaptic receptors, which are located some distance from sites of NO synthesis. In addition, nNOS-containing neurons actively participate in the rostral path of neuroblast migration, which involves new synaptic connections and influences neurogenesis [39]. Astrocyte migration is also regulated by the release of NO under the actions of inducible nitric oxide synthase (iNOS). NO is also recognized as critical for the formation of synapses and the growth of nerve fibers [40].

Deficits in synaptic plasticity are increasingly recognized as causes of memory loss in AD [41]. NO is produced by NOS through NMDAR-mediated calcium input. NO signaling comes into play in neurodegenerative diseases via the generation of reactive nitrogen species and cGMP signaling cascades. NO also exerts neuroprotective effects, as shown in AD mouse models, by reducing cell loss and Tau pathology [42]. In AD models, NO has shown to be altered through various mechanisms. For example, the NMDAR-mediated calcium entry that activates NOS is enhanced by abnormal ryanodine receptor-(RyR-) mediated calcium-induced calcium release. NOS and RyR protein levels are also increased in both AD mouse models and human AD brains. In AD mice, at the presynaptic level, these conditions increasing NO levels take place alongside excessive hippocampal synaptic depression. These deficits occur when homeostasis is placed at risk, such as in the presence of reduced RyR-calcium release. Consequently, the hippocampal network and cognitive function are not normal, though they appear to be so [43].

In a study on 3×-Tg-AD mice, the presynaptic terminals have shown to be the primary site of NO regulation, with increased evoked and spontaneous vesicle release, as determined by paired-pulse facilitation assays and spontaneous vesicle-release properties [44]. Moreover, NO modifies the magnitude of vesicular release by transforming spare vesicles into easily releasable vesicles [45]. In addition, NO can increase the opening of RyR channels, possibly by means of S-nitrosylation. The opposite interactions between augmented RyR-calcium signaling and enhanced nNOS expression in AD neurons can sustain an increased NO production or synthesis and also strengthen the presynaptic gain. At the postsynaptic level, the neuroprotective characteristics of NO become evident by inhibiting the excessive NMDAR-induced calcium influx and excitotoxicity via S-nitrosylation of the NR2A subunit of the NMDA receptor. At the same time, apoptosis is decreased through the S-nitrosylation of caspase-3, -8, and -9. The enhanced nNOS activity and NO levels in AD brains might be neuroprotective, as proven by the selectively preserved NOS-positive neurons in AD. Hence, continuous increases in NO exert harmful effects, such as oxidative stress, the shredder loss of synaptic function, and apoptosis [46].

All in all, the NO up-regulation or down-regulation may result in neuropsychiatric conditions, and its improvement may restore synaptic plasticity and neuronal function. Understanding the specific molecular mechanisms maintaining these effects can give some light as to identify ways to treat these neuropsychiatric conditions [47]. Particularly, pathological deficits in NO signaling have been reported in corticostriatal circuits in Huntington's disease (HD). Studies indicate that deficits in cortical and striatal nNOS activity and nitrergic transmission may contribute to the progression of corticostriatal pathway dysfunction observed in HD. In this pathology, medium-sized spiny neurons (MSNs) projecting to the external globus pallidus appear to preferentially degenerate as a consequence of accumulation of the abnormal huntingtin protein. What is interesting is that cortical stimulation increases striatal NOS activity by means of a NMDA and dopamine D1 receptor-dependent mechanism. Thus, studies on nNOS knockout mice have proven that striatal MSNs are significantly less sensitive to cortical drive when compared with wild-type controls, indicating that NO signaling plays a critical role in maintaining corticostriatal transmission [48]. Therefore, deficiencies in nNOS activity and NO signaling reported in HD could be associated with decreased excitatory corticostriatal transmission and motor dysfunction. From this concluding remark, it is likely that HD patients might benefit from pharmacotherapies aimed to favor nitrergic signaling and corticostriatal transmission.

Conversely, the protective effect of NMDA antagonists in conditions of *in vivo* cerebral ischemia supports that influx of Ca^{2+} through NMDA-receptor channels constitute the main driver of glutamate neurotoxicity, a mechanism being of pathological importance. Studies on the role of NO in NMDA-mediated neurodegeneration have given some light with the use of mice lacking individual NOSs subjected to ischemia. For instance, it has been found that nNOS contributed to the early damage, whereas endothelial NOS (eNOS) was protective, reflecting its relevance in cerebral blood flow and, likely, in inhibiting both leucocyte adhesion to the endothelium and platelet aggregation [49]. Reduced synthesis and availability of eNO may contribute to the development of dementia by favoring the onset and progression of atherosclerosis, vasoconstriction, and impaired cerebral blood flow regulation. Furthermore, the inducible isoform of NOS (iNOS) that starts to be expressed in the following days to an ischemic event appeared to provide additional damage. iNOS is expressed in macrophages and glial cells in response to pro-inflammatory cytokines or endotoxin. In the brain, widespread expression of iNOS is pathologic and has been observed in neurological diseases, such as multiple sclerosis, stroke, and AD. Increased NO production and iNOS expression have been observed after experimental and clinical traumatic brain injury (TBI). iNOS knock-out mice showed reduction in infarct volume and motor deficits after focal ischemia compared with wild-type mice. In an exploratory phase II study trial, TBI patients treated with the most selective inhibitor of human iNOS reported to date showed significant improvement in clinical outcome [50]. These studies suggested a neuroprotective effect of iNOS inhibition after TBI.

5. Astrocyte involvement—astroglial CB1 receptors

Astrocytes are the most abundant glial cell population in the brain [51]. One of the most intriguing features of astrocytes is the control of synaptic plasticity and memory functions. Astrocytes contribute in shaping different types of synaptic plasticity that challenges the generation of experimental models enabling the distinction between the neuronal contribution and the astroglial contribution in the control of a given function [52].

The finding of a large number of astrocytes and increased expression of the α7 nAChRs subunit on these cells in hippocampus and temporal cortex of sporadic AD patients have suggested an involvement of the astrocytic α7 nAChRs in the metabolism of Aβ and a relationship with the amyloid cascade [53]. It has been proven that Aβ, at physiological levels, controls synaptic activity and acts as a positive or negative regulator post-synaptically. In fact, Aβ either activates or inhibits α7 nAChRs in a dose-dependent manner. In the healthy brain, Aβ enhances spontaneous astrocyte calcium transients, regulating neuron-glia signaling in a nAChR-dependent manner [54]. On the other hand, Aβ accumulation increases astrocytic α7 nAChRs expression and subsequently increases intracellular calcium released from intracellular stores contributing to a number of inflammatory cascades.

The nAChRs from astrocytes can be activated by the transmitters released from presynaptic terminals or neurotransmitters located in the interstitial space [52]. For instance, the nAChRs agonist acetylcholine elevates intracellular calcium in astrocytes, stimulating the release of glutamate gliotransmitter and consequently the NMDA receptor-dependent currents in neurons. It results in an increase of the efficient synaptic transmission and strength. This mechanism explains the Aβ-induced hippocampal LTP. Then, Aβ-α7 nAChRs interaction increases astrocytic activity to induce glutamate gliotransmission which contributes to synaptic plasticity and cognition [55]. However, pathological concentrations of Aβ, as occurred in AD, induces LTD as Aβ oligomers-induced glutamate release from astrocytes causes excitotoxic damage and synaptic loss in neurons. In essence, pathological levels of Aβ cause α7 nAChR-induced gliotransmission dysregulation leading to increased excitability within the hippocampal neural network [56]. What is more, endogenous stimulation of α7 nAChRs on astrocytes causes expression of further AMPA receptors post-synaptically at glutamatergic synapses of neurons. Consequently, the ratio of AMPA-evoked synaptic currents increases.

There is evidence that GABA is abundantly produced and released by activated astrocytes. A non-physiological increase in tonic GABA release from reactive astrocytes in the hippocampus may be directly responsible for the memory impairment in AD. It has been shown that alterations of kynurenic acid, an astrocyte-derived antagonist of the α7 nAChRs, are associated with the impairment of the cognitive function in AD patients. In fact, kynurenic acid at low concentrations inhibits GABAergic neurotransmission triggered by α7 nAChRs activation [57]. Therefore, prevention of GABAergic neurotransmission by α7 nAChRs inhibition through kynurenic acid may protect against AD.

The α7-specific agonists decrease IL-6 production in cell lines derived from astrocytes. Conversely, internalization of these receptors in astrocytes by binding to α7-specific antibodies could stimulate IL-6 production. The α7 nAChRs internalization might provoke neuroinflammation within the brain by inducing IL-6 production in astrocytes. Furthermore, evidence shows that treatment with different α7 nAChRs agonists prevent neuroinflammation in AD-affected brains and suppress elevated levels of astrocyte-related pro-inflammatory cytokines, such as TNF-α [58].

Microglia play different roles in the healthy brain which include neuronal synapse monitoring, phagocytosis of neuronal debris, and cell migration as well as proliferation. Microglia show a typical resting phenotype in the healthy CNS, becoming activated in response to excessive neuronal activity during neurochemical or electrically stimulations. It has been shown that increased activation of astrocytic α4β2 and α7 nAChRs drives the expression of glial cell-derived neurotrophic factor (GDNF) [59]. Astrocyte-derived GDNF binds to GDNF family receptor alpha1 (GFRα1) and activates intracellular signaling pathways that lead to inhibition of microglial activation and protection of neurons from neurodegeneration [60].

The astroglial type-1-cannabinoid (CB1) receptor signaling recently emerged as the mediator of several forms of synaptic plasticity associated to important cognitive functions [61]. The presence of CB1 and type-2 (CB2) receptors in astrocytes was first described in human and rodent primary cultures. Particularly, CB1 receptors are mainly located at presynaptic terminals of different types of neurons, inhibiting neurotransmitter release. Although the signaling of CB1 receptors in astrocytes has been partially investigated, it has been suggested that they are able to couple to different intracellular signaling pathways in this type of cells, therefore providing high adaptability to endocannabinoid-mediated responses in these cells. The first endocannabinoid identified was arachidonoyl-ethanolamide, known as anandamide [62]. Arachidonoyl-ethanolamide mimics the cannabinoid "tetrad" effects (i.e., hypolocomotion, antinociception, catalepsy, and hypothermia) in rodents. The second discovered endocannabinoid, 2-arachidonoyl-glycerol (2-AG) is considered as the main effector of most of the CB1 receptor-mediated endogenous regulation of synaptic transmission. Endocannabinoids' precursors are located in cell membranes and their transformation into actual endocannabinoids is thought to mainly occur in an activity-dependent manner. Endocannabinoids are likely produced, mobilized, and degraded by astrocytes *in vivo*, suggesting the presence of an astroglial autocrine and/or paracrine endocannabinoid signaling.

Astrocytic processes express transporters GLT-1 and GLAST for glutamate, participating in the rapid removal of glutamate released into the synaptic cleft, which is essential for both the termination of synaptic transmission and maintenance of physiological neuronal excitability. Since increased stimulation of glutamate receptors is highly toxic for neurons, glutamate uptake by astrocytes is crucial for protecting neurons against excitotoxicity. In this regard, it has been observed that pharmacological blockade of CB1 receptors reduces epileptiform discharges of hippocampal slices through a direct control on astrocytic calcium signaling, suggesting that over-activation of astroglial CB1 receptors might promote the maintenance of brain excitotoxicity [61].

Intriguingly, whereas CB1 receptors on glutamatergic neurons have been found to reduce glutamate release and excitoxicity, astroglial CB1 receptors have been shown to promote astroglial-dependent activation of glutamatergic transmission [63]. These potentially opposite effects at neurons or astroglial cells might indicate the complexity in the regulation of excitatory output by the endocannabinoid system.

However, arachidonoyl-ethanolamide has shown to reverse AMPA-induced neurotoxicity and down-regulation of GLT-1 and GLAST (glutamate transporters) mRNA in cultures of mouse astrocyte and in the spinal cord of a mouse model of multiple sclerosis via CB1 receptor [64]. Thus, the role of astroglial CB1 receptors in the regulation of excitatory amino acids in the context of excitotoxic processes might depend on the conditions of the brain circuits involved and the specific activation of the endocannabinoid system at different sites. It might be hypothesized that astroglial CB1 receptors might exert a bidirectional control of excitatory transmission and excitotoxicity [61].

The role of astroglial CB1 receptors in the modulation of excitatory transmission in the hippocampus was first reported by Navarrete and Araque [65]. They found that hippocampal astrocytes express functional CB1 receptors that increase intracellular Ca^{2+} levels in astrocytes following electrical stimulation of adjacent neurons. CB1 receptor-dependent increase of intracellular Ca^{2+} levels in astrocytes requires activation of PLC, suggesting that the interaction of CB1 receptors with the $G\alpha q$ protein subunit may be favored in astrocytes as compared to neurons. Astroglial CB1 receptors activation is necessary for NMDA receptor-mediated neuronal excitability evoked by astrocyte Ca^{2+} elevations, suggesting their importance for astrocyte-neuron excitatory signaling. However, these results do not characterize neither the endogenous NMDA receptor agonist implicated in this process nor the cellular origin and identity of the released eCBs that act at astroglial CB1 receptors in these conditions. Astroglial CB1 receptors mediate heterosynaptic potentiation at excitatory CA3-CA1 synapses in a Group I mGluR-dependent fashion. Importantly, this phenomenon coexists with depolarization-induced suppression of excitation (DSE, short-term inhibition of excitatory transmission) mediated by neuronal CB1 receptors at homosynaptic connections [66].

Finally, astroglial CB1 receptors mediate spike timing-dependent LTD (tLTD) in the neocortex. tLTD is induced by paired stimulations of the pre- and postsynaptic elements, leading to a reduction of presynaptic release of glutamate. CB1 receptor-dependent tLTD has been also described at cortico-striatal synapses and may imply astroglial CB1 signaling as well. This form of synaptic plasticity has been associated to the neuronal coding of sensory experiences *in vivo*. Interestingly, one of the major consequences of exogenous cannabinoids administration, including THC, is an alteration of perception, but little is known about the mechanisms underlying these effects [67]. Therefore, it is possible that the overstimulation of CB1 receptors impairs sensory functions by a deregulation of tLTD.

6. The microtubule-associated neuronal protein Tau

The neuronal cytoskeleton is the major intracellular structure that determines the morphology of neurons and plays a critical role in the development of the nervous system, neuronal plasticity, and neurodegenerative diseases [68]. In particular, changes in microtubule (MT) dynamics are involved not only in axon formation and axonal sprouting but also in mediating structural and functional changes of dendritic spines, which represent the major site of excitatory postsynaptic input [69].

MT dynamics are regulated by several factors affecting the assembly state of this polymer. MT-associated proteins (MAPs) promote MT nucleation and elongation in a compartment-specific manner and are also subject to regulation by posttranslational modification [69]. Tau is of particular importance since it becomes enriched in the axonal compartment during neuronal development and redistributes to the somato-dendritic compartment in a state of hyperphosphorylation during neurodegenerative pathologies such as AD and other tauopathies [70]. Strikingly, acute or chronic knockdown of Tau does not appear to affect MT stability and organization or the overall structure of a neuron to a major extent. This feature raises the question whether Tau possesses activities beyond its direct role in regulating axonal MT polymerization, which is altered in AD and other tauopathies. In this regard, Tau is an intrinsically disordered protein, which interacts with different partners. Tau stands out for its structural plasticity allowing it to react quickly in response to changes in their environment by posttranslational modifications [71]. Then, Tau may affect various signaling and regulatory processes dependent on its modification, thereby regulating the function and plasticity of neurons during learning, memory, and degenerative processes.

In order to make a functional assessment of Tau role with regard to neuronal activity and network properties, several electrophysiological studies have been performed using Tau knock-out (KO) mice or Tau knockdown experiments. Complete absence of Tau or a decrease in the amount of Tau on neuronal activity has been studied by recordings from individual cortical neurons as well as from intact neuronal circuits in acutely isolated tissue slices. The focus in most studies was placed on the influence of Tau on LTP or LTD generation in the hippocampus both being established experimental paradigms of synaptic plasticity underlying learning and memory formation. Cantero et al. [72] has studied the involvement of Tau in shaping electrophysiological properties of neural oscillations in different neocortical regions and hippocampus during spontaneous exploratory motor behavior of 4 month old mice. They observed a significant slowdown of the hippocampal theta rhythm, which is known to play a crucial role in learning and memory function. Furthermore, they found decreased levels of gamma long-range synchronization in the KO animals, while power and peak frequency in the gamma band oscillations (30–80 Hz) recorded from neocortex and hippocampus remained unchanged. As a result, it was hypothesized that the lack of physiologically phosphorylated Tau during early stages of development may influence the maturation of parvalbumin-containing interneurons affecting the spatiotemporal structure of long-range gamma synchronization between hippocampus and neocortex.

It was recently demonstrated that Tau exerts an important mediatory role in regulating the interaction between protein kinase C binding protein 1 and GluA2, a molecular mechanism fundamental to AMPA receptor internalization [73]. Biochemical and electrophysiological assays have allowed to show that specific phosphorylation at S396 of Tau is related to and required for LTD. In addition, the absence of Tau led to the reversion of deficiencies in spatial memory, pointing out a relevant role of Tau in hippocampal LTD. Thus, Tau seems to be decisively involved in the maintenance of physiological synaptic transmission and synaptic plasticity.

For many years, in terms of location, Tau has been considered to be an exclusively intracellular protein. However, Tau can be released from neurons and it has been found in the cerebrospinal fluid of AD patients. This feature may affect network functions by directly influencing the activity of multiple neurons. Stimulation of neuronal activity can induce Tau release from healthy cortical neurons, suggesting that Tau secretion is a physiological process [74]. *In vivo* microdialysis has proven that increasing neuronal activity raises the level of extracellular Tau. The elimination rate of Tau from the extracellular space in the brain is slow suggesting that Tau can be present for long times outside of neurons and influence other cells. Extracellular Tau has a reduced phosphorylation state and is enriched in C-terminally truncated forms. Besides, it has been demonstrated that a Tau fragment resulting from the cleavage through the effector caspase-3 exhibits enhanced secretion [75]. It is not yet clear in which form Tau is present in the extracellular space and how it potentially influences other neurons. Extracellular Tau might affect network functions by acting on other cells through receptor-mediated mechanisms. Alternatively, extracellular Tau might be taken up by other neurons and modulate their signaling cascades. Several studies have reported uptake of Tau aggregates and oligomers, which may cause network damage by propagation of protein abnormalities. For instance, it has been suggested a prion-like spreading of a pathogenic misfolded Tau in a deterministic manner to distinct brain regions [76]. However, it is not clear whether or not extracellular soluble Tau is internalized by neurons at physiological conditions. Application of exogenous Tau from cerebral cortex of AD brain evoked a strong LTP inhibition at CA3-CA1 synapses in hippocampal brain slices being elicited by theta burst stimulation. Moreover, a short exposure to oligomers, but not monomers, of extracellular recombinant human Tau causes a concentration-dependent impairment of LTP in the CA3-CA1 pathway and memory formation [77]. These effects were reproduced both by Tau oligomers from AD human specimens, as well as those produced in mice overexpressing the human Tau. *In vitro* conditions has evidenced that oligomerized Tau passes the cell membrane and is internalized by neurons. However, it is unclear whether extracellular Tau acts in these experiments through receptor-mediated mechanisms or after internalization.

With all of it, it appears clear that Tau exerts systemic effects and modulates network functions both in the CNS and the peripheral nervous system. Consequently, changes in the Tau level will produce various side effects. Though most available data are still controversial at length, general trends begin to become apparent from several experimental approaches. The course of motor impairments as a consequence of reduced Tau levels at advanced age might be caused by an impact on the peripheral motor system. Mild cognitive and memory deficits and a disruption of physiological synaptic transmission and synaptic plasticity have been repeatedly reported. Even posttranslational modifications of Tau possessing pathologic effect may serve protective functions for synapses, which would be impaired in circumstances of Tau depletion. Experiments with hibernating animals have rendered evidence for a protective function of Tau phosphorylation, providing a striking model for extreme plasticity, as numerous synaptic contacts are lost during hibernation and regenerated in a brief period of time after animal awakening. In these animals, a physiologically adaptive process associated with synaptic plasticity seems to be supported by a reversible hyperphosphorylation of soluble Tau [78].

Furthermore, a small amount of Tau has been localized and accumulated in the nuclear compartment, in both the soluble and chromatin-bound fractions. A putative role of Tau in both nucleolar organization and DNA damage protection and chromosome stability have been proposed, since wild-type Tau prevents DNA damage under oxidative stress or hyperthermic conditions. Recently, it has been observed that promoting Tau nuclear translocation and accumulation, by Tau overexpression or disengagement from MTs, enhances the expression of the vesicular glutamate transporter VGluT1 [79], a disease-fundamental gene directly involved in glutamatergic transmission. Significantly, the P301L mutation in Tau gene, linked to frontotemporal dementia FTDP-17 [80], disturbs this mechanism leading to a function loss. This fact demonstrates a direct physiological role of Tau on modulating gene expression, particularly the expression of the vesicular glutamate transporter VGluT1, which is known to be strongly upregulated in early phases of tauopathies. Thus, alterations of this mechanism may be at the basis of the onset of neurodegeneration.

Taken together, though most current approaches to target Tau are based on its actions on MTs and are aimed at counteracting the aggregation of its soluble pool, unlinked functions of Tau to its MT-binding properties have been suggested lately. Therefore, in view of the evidence supporting considerable modulatory and potentially protective functions of Tau at physiological conditions, the strategies aimed at modulating the amount and modification of Tau should be carefully taken into consideration when planning Tau-based therapies.

7. The signaling pathway of the Wnt protein family

In humans, Wnts are a family of secreted glycolipoproteins (19 members) that are evolutionarily conserved [81]. Wnts are essential for axon pathfinding, dendritic development, and the formation and function of synapses [82]. The contribution of Wnts to synapse development in different model systems has been supported widely [83].

Several Wnt proteins (Wnt7a, Wnt5a, and Wnt3a) that signal through different receptors promote pre-synaptic differentiation [84]. Besides, Wnts signaling promotes excitatory synapse formation and spine growth [85]. Unlike Wnt7a, Wnt5a promotes inhibitory post-synaptic assembly by increasing GABA$_A$ receptor clustering and enhancing the amplitude of inhibitory postsynaptic currents [86]. Members of the Wnt family might regulate excitatory and inhibitory post-synaptic properties, differentially. Moreover, Wnts act bidirectionally to promote the assembly of both sides of the synapse [84].

Regulation of synaptic transmission by Wnt proteins has been demonstrated by electrophysiological recordings. Members of the Wnt family can modulate neurotransmission pre-synaptically and post-synaptically [84]. For instance, gain of function of Wnt7a has shown to promote transmitter release in cultured neurons. Post-synaptically, Wnt7a enhances synaptic strength by increasing the number of AMPA receptors at the post-synaptic membrane in hippocampal neurons and Wnt5a potentiates post-synaptic NMDAR-mediated currents through RoR2 receptors in hippocampal neurons.

Members of the Wnt family are regulated by neuronal activity. Thus, neuronal activity modulates the mRNA and protein levels of Wnts and their receptors in different model systems. Wnt blockade completely abolishes activity-mediated synapse formation in cultured neurons [87]. Blockade of endogenous Wnt proteins, with secreted frizzled-related proteins (Sfrps), severely impairs LTP [88]. Conversely, addition of Wnt proteins can facilitate LTP [89].

Research is been currently focused on identifying the mechanisms by which Wnts modulate LTP. In this regard, Wnt5a has been shown to regulate NMDAR-mediated synaptic transmission in acute hippocampal slices [89]. However, it does not affect endogenous synaptic AMPAR localization or dendritic spine size in hippocampal cultured neurons [88]. Then, it is suggested that Wnt5a may contribute to later stages of LTP.

Endogenous Wnt signaling is required for structural and functional plasticity during LTP as it has been demonstrated. A study shows that Wnt7a/b regulate the early stages of NMDAR-dependent LTP [88]. Acute blockade of endogenous Wnts with Sfrps attenuates LTP induced by stimulating acute hippocampal slices at high frequency or LTP induced by glycine application in hippocampal neurons. Changes in dendritic spine structure, augmented synaptic strength, and synaptic localization of AMPA receptors are inhibited in the presence of Sfrps during LTP. Intriguingly, gain of function via single-particle tracking and super-ecliptic pHluorin-tagged AMPA receptors in hippocampal neurons has proven that Wnt7a quickly enhances dendritic spine growth, recruitment of synaptic AMPA receptors, and synaptic strength, similar to the early phases of LTP [88].

A proper balance between canonical and non-canonical Wnt signaling might determine whether synapses are lost or only their function is affected [84]. A mouse model characterized by a Wnt deficiency in the adult brain has demonstrated that Wnt proteins constitute a requirement for synapse stability and synaptic plasticity [90]. Transgenic mice expressing the Wnt antagonist Dickkopf-1 (Dkk1) protein in hippocampus display a loss of excitatory synapses, altered LTP, enhanced LTD, and deficits in long-term memory [91]. Acute blockade of endogenous Wnts by Sfrps does not affect the number of excitatory synapses but inhibits LTP induction. This is not due to acute versus long-term exposure to Wnt antagonists, as Dkk1 also rapidly induces synapse loss in mature neurons [92]. Both antagonists have a different mechanism of action. While Sfrps inhibits Wnt function by means of binding to Wnt proteins, Dkk1 affects a canonical Wnt signaling pathway by blocking the low density lipoprotein receptor-related protein 6 (LRP6), an essential Wnt co-receptor.

Growing evidence suggests that deficient Wnt signaling affects synaptic integrity in the adult brain. In AD, particularly, decreased levels of Wnt signaling could weaken synaptic function resulting in the subsequent degeneration and loss of synapses characteristic of this condition. Expression of the endogenous Wnt antagonist Dkk1 is increased in the brain of AD patients. On other hand, Aß quickly induces Dkk1 expression and blockade of Dkk1 protects synapses from Aß [92]. Besides, a variant of LRP6 has been linked to late onset AD [93] and deletion of LRP6 magnifies pathology in an AD mouse model [94]. These findings along with those obtained from mice expressing Dkk1 [91] demonstrate that deficits in Wnt signaling affect synaptic integrity in the adult brain. In AD, diminished levels of Wnt signaling could mine synaptic function leading to the subsequent degeneration and synapse loss which is characteristic of this condition. Reactivation of Wnt signaling might restore connectivity after substantial synapse degeneration. In fact, the ceasing of Dkk1 expression in transgenic mice that express Dkk1 fully restores the structural and functional plasticity and hippocampal-dependent memory [91]. Together, these studies prove the regenerative capacity of neurons in the adult hippocampus to assemble synapses within functional circuits after degeneration.

8. Extracellular vesicles in the intercellular communication

In the CNS, extracellular vesicles (EVs) have emerged as key players in the intercellular communication that underlies physiological processes such as synaptic plasticity, maintenance of myelination, and neuronal and glial response to brain injury. EVs are secreted membrane-enclosed 'packages' that contain cytosolic proteins, membrane proteins, mRNAs, noncoding RNAs, and even DNA [95].

In order to modulate synaptic plasticity, neuronal EVs can transfer cargo to other neurons. It has been suggested an uptake of neuronal EVs by microglia to enhance microglial pruning of synapses. Moreover, increased astrocytic uptake of glutamate may result from internalization of neuronal EVs into astrocytes. In turn, EVs from astrocytes have been shown to contain cargo-mediating neuroprotection under neuronal stress. Oligodendrocyte-derived EVs increase neuronal firing mediate as well as neuronal stress resilience [96]. Moreover, oligodendrocyte-derived EVs may behave as auto-inhibitors in expansion of myelin. As for microglial EVs, they may modulate neuronal firing, and also propagate inflammation and destabilize synapses in a CNS injury setting. In terms of neurodegenerative diseases, EVs are involved in both the spreading and clearance of neurotoxic protein aggregates [97]. EVs have also been shown to cross the blood-brain barrier particularly under inflammatory conditions, enabling molecular crosstalk between brain cells and the periphery [98].

The coupling of neuronal EV release to synaptic activity could be functionally relevant for plasticity-associated processes. For instance, activity-dependent disposal or transfer of AMPA receptor components, which have been shown to flow throughout EVs, may constitute a mechanism for the adjustment of synaptic strength [99]. Moreover, it has been suggested that neuronal EVs act as trans-synaptic carriers of signaling proteins involved in synaptic plasticity. In a series of *in vivo* studies at the *Drosophila* neuromuscular junction, it has been shown that the Wnt-family signaling protein Wingless was protected driving toward EVs by the trafficking protein Evi/Wntless for trans-synaptic transport and hampering this trafficking impaired synaptic bouton formation [100]. In the same model system, synaptotagmin 4 has been found to drive on EVs from the presynaptic motor neuron to the postsynaptic muscle, and this directional transport was fundamental for activity-dependent growth of presynaptic structures.

Plasticity-associated local protein synthesis at synapses appears to be affected by the activity-dependent trafficking of specific RNAs into EVs. In one study, depolarization of differentiated neuroblasts has been found to be correlated with a depletion of specific miRNAs from neurites, associated with an enhancement of a specific subset of these miRNAs in EVs. Furthermore, neuronal EVs have been recently shown to package mRNA in association with the activity-regulated cytoskeleton-associated protein (Arc), described as a master regulator of synaptic plasticity [101]. Arc appeared to self-assemble into capsids as if it were a viral group-specific antigen (Gag) protein, encapsulating its own mRNA or other highly abundant mRNAs, and trafficking between cells by means of EVs. The blockage of Arc trafficking from presynaptic terminals to the postsynaptic muscle, at the Drosophila neuromuscular junction, caused aberrations in synapse maturation and activity-dependent plasticity [102]. Therefore, Arc capsid-containing EVs may constitute a retrovirus-like mechanism for trans-synaptic transfer of at least Arc mRNA during processes associated with synaptic plasticity. The biological origin and composition of Arc-containing EVs, as well as the scope of the EV-associated Arc transport in the mammalian brain, have yet to be studied in the future.

It is intriguing that neuronal EVs can also transfer cargo to other cells in the brain, modulating their behavior with a potential impact on synaptic activity. One study found that the uptake of neuronal miR-124a-carrying EVs into astrocytes was correlated with overexpression of excitatory amino acid transporter 2/glutamate transporter-1 (EAAT2/GLT1), which could modulate synaptic activity via an increased uptake of glutamate into perisynaptic astrocytes [103]. Moreover, EVs from differentiated PC12 cells seemed to promote microglial phagocytosis of degenerating neurites by means of increasing the microglial expression of complement component 3 (C3), a factor associated with synaptic pruning. The release of EVs from active neurons could thereby serve to the removal of less functional synapses during developmental or learning-associated remodeling of neuronal connections, although validation of this finding is warranted in at least primary neurons.

With regard to glial EVs, they have been described to provide neurons with support and feedback on synaptic activity. And so, for example, oligodendrocytes contain multivesicular endosomes at sites near the axonal surface, and secrete EVs particularly in response to glutamate. While microglia appeared to degrade oligodendrocyte-derived EVs, neuronal internalization of these EVs led to functional cargo retrieval along with an increase in neuronal firing rate and modified gene expression of several plasticity-related targets, such as VGF nerve growth factor inducible and BDNF [104]. Microglial microvesicles (MVs), for its part, released in response to ATP and increased excitatory neurotransmission through stimulation of neuronal sphingolipid metabolism and a consequent increase in the presynaptic release of neurotransmitters. The functionality of the MVs seemed to depend on a lipid or a surface component since sheared MVs retained the functionality [105]. In another study, microglial EVs have shown to carry the active endocannabinoid N-arachidonoylethanolamine on their surface, which bound to presynaptic type 1 cannabinoid receptors, and thereby decreased the release of the neurotransmitter GABA. Overall, glial EVs seem to influence both excitatory and inhibitory neurotransmission, providing regulatory feedback particularly on pre-synaptic activity [95].

As remarkable, EVs have emerged as possible therapeutic agents in inflammation-mediated demyelinating diseases, such as multiple sclerosis (MS). Increasing evidence suggests that EVs display anti-inflammatory properties, reducing the number of activated inflammatory microglial cells, supporting oligo-dendrocytes and protecting neurons. A very recent study illustrates a putative therapeutically role for EVs. Intravenously administered EVs derived from mesen-chymal stem cells (MSCs) from human adipose tissue might mediate recovery in Theiler's murine encephalomyelitis virus (TMEV)-induced demyelinating disease, a progressive model of MS [106]. Intravenous EV administration in SJL/J mice improved motor deficits, lowered brain atrophy, enhanced cell proliferation in the subventricular zone, and decreased inflammatory infiltrates in the spinal cord of animals infected with TMEV. In addition, EV treatment was capable of modulating neuroinflammation, given glial fibrillary acidic protein and Iba-1 staining were reduced in the brain, whereas the expression of myelin was increased. Modifica-tions of morphology in microglial cells from the spinal cord may indicate that EVs also modulate the activation state of microglia. EV administration attenuates motor deficits through immunomodulatory actions, diminishing brain atrophy and pro-moting remyelination.

So far, there is no evidence regarding the therapeutic potential of EVs during the neurodegenerative phase of MS. Further studies are necessary to establish EV delivery as a possible therapy for the neurodegenerative phase of MS.

9. Estrogen involvement in non-reproductive functions

Estrogens from neural origin are involved in a variety of non-reproductive functions including regulation of neurogenesis, neuronal development, synaptic transmission, and plasticity in brain regions not directly related with the control of reproduction [107]. Estrogens regulate the expression of genes for various specific subtypes of dopamine (DA) receptors and 5-HT receptors in a region-specific manner to contribute to behavioral responses to changes of the internal and external environment.

DA neurotransmission of the ventral tegmental area (VTA)-nucleus accumbens (NAc) pathway associated with motivation is modulated by estrogens, which results in functional differences of the mesolimbic dopaminergic pathway and explains numerous sex differences in reward processing and related behavior described in human and animal studies [108]. Generally, increased circulating levels of estrogens in rodents, either during their estrous cycles or by estrogen treatment, have shown to contribute to elevated dopaminergic signaling. Estrogens influence manifold aspects of dopaminergic neurotransmission both presynaptically and postsynaptically, including: (a) DA synthesis, release, and degradation; (b) presyn-aptic and postsynaptic receptors; and (c) DA transporters that uptake DA from the synapse to terminate DA neurotransmission. Nuclear and membrane-associated estrogen receptors (ERs) may constitute the mechanisms by which estrogens affect the dopaminergic system. Precisely, ERs are distributed in dopaminergic pathways involved in reward, what is pertinent to the effects of estrogens on the CNS reward system [109]. In male mice, dopaminergic projections from the VTA to the ventral caudate express the ERβ isoform, while dopaminergic projections to the dorsal caudate do not. Dopaminergic projections to the basolateral amygdala also express ERβ. Estrogens also act rapidly through membrane-associated ERs on dopaminergic neurons in the striatum to affect DA release. Estrogens increase the activity of the tyrosine hydroxylase (TH) and thus DA synthesis in the NAc by means of both nuclear ERs and membrane ER; induce presynaptic DA release in the striatum; and decrease DA turnover in the NAc and reduce degradation of DA so that DA remains longer at the synapse [108].

Estrogens upregulate the expression and activity of tryptophan hydroxylase (TPH) to increase 5-HT biosynthesis. Estrogen administration has been found to increase the TPH mRNA level [110]. In ovariectomized (OVX) guinea pigs, estrogen treatment alone increases the protein expression of TPH at the dorsal raphe nucleus (DRN). Surprisingly, while treatment with estrogen alone increases levels of TPH mRNA and TPH protein, it does not modify 5-HT content; rather, the treatment combining estrogen plus progesterone enhances 5-HT levels at both the DRN and the projected medial basal hypothalamus in guinea pigs [111]. Thus, there is a disparity in the sex hormone regulation of TPH mRNA and TPH protein levels versus 5-HT production in estrogen-treated animals, likely due to activity of TPH that is regulated by means of phosphorylation by protein kinase A (PKA) [112]. Since only phosphorylated TPH possesses catalytic activity, progesterone treatment might increase PKA expression and activity of TPH. After loss of ovarian function in many women, there may be an adjustment in the serotonergic neurons so that TPH protein levels recover. This also may indicate that the decline in TPH expression is a potential point of vulnerability in pre- and postmenopausal women who experience mental disorders such as depression related to the decreased level of 5-HT.

Estrogens regulate the 5-HT receptors, 5-HT2A and 2C, which display classic features of G protein-coupled receptors. The 5-HT2A receptor has been associated with suicide and depression, and its mRNAs are found in brain areas fundamental for the mood control, mental state, and cognition [113]. In humans, 5-HT2A receptor mRNA is found in the cortex and hippocampus, but not in the DRN, striatum, substantia nigra, or cerebellum [114]. Estrogens increase 5-HT2A receptor mRNA and binding site densities in the male rat brain. Healthy men have shown significantly higher levels of 5-HT2A receptor binding capacity than healthy women in the frontal and cingulate cortices, according to determinations by PET and radiotracer 18F-labeled altanserin [115]. Human studies suggest that estrogens increase 5-HT2A binding in higher forebrain regions.

The NAc receives major inputs from the amygdala and projects to the cortex and hypothalamus. These regions are fundamental for the cognitive function, emotion, mental state, mood, and neuroendocrine control. Thus, increase in 5-HT2A receptor densities by estrogen stimulation in these stated regions would control behavior and mood. A single administration of estradiol to OVX rats induces a significant increase in 5-HT2A receptor labeling in the NAc, the amygdala, DRN, anterior frontal, anterior cingulate, and primary olfactory cortex [116]. Moreover, concomitantly with the spontaneous estrogen-induced LH surge, 5-HT2A receptor densities increase compared to diestrous females or males in the frontal and cingulate cortex, olfactory tubercle and NAc. OVX produces a reduction of 5-HT2A receptor mRNA and protein levels, and long-term estrogen replacement reverses this effect in the frontal cortex [117]. The receptor 5-HT2C, a relevant contributor of many psychiatric and neurological disorders, is the most prominent 5-HT receptor subtype in the rat brain. 5-HT2C mRNA and protein are found in discrete regions of the rat brain. In the primate hypothalamus, dense populations of 5-HT2C mRNA-labeled cells are found in the anterior hypothalamus, periventricular nuclei, ventromedial nucleus, dorsal hypothalamic area, lateral hypothalamus, arcuate nucleus, and infundibular nucleus [118].

Estrogens regulate 5-HT auto-inhibition via the 5-HT1A auto-receptor. The 5-HT1A auto-receptor suppresses 5-HT synthesis by inhibiting firing of serotonergic neurons at the DRN and median raphe and inhibiting 5-HT release in the hippocampus [119]. Therefore, the blockage of 5-HT1A receptors results in an antidepressant-like activity. Estrogen treatment lowers the 5-HT1A mRNA level in the dentate gyrus, CA2 region of the hippocampus, and DRN of OVX rats and in the DRN and median raphe of castrated rhesus monkeys, according to measurement by in situ hybridization. The5-HT1A auto-receptor is linked to an inhibitory G protein of the Gi/o/zfamily [120].

Estrogen treatment reduces 5-HT uptake to presynaptic cells by means of decreasing gene expression, translation, protein phosphorylation, trafficking, and stability of the serotonin transporter (SERT) [121]. Estrogens reduce SERT mRNA signal in the DRN of castrated rhesus monkeys treated with estrogen compared to the castrated control group and decrease [^{3}H]-paroxetine binding, a selective indicator of 5-HT reuptake sites, in the hippocampus of estrogen-treated rats. Acute estrogen administration decreases SERT mRNA levels and 5-HT1A mRNA levels and binding. Thus, estrogen replacement therapy in postmenopausal women might decrease expression of the SERT gene and SERT protein [107]; thus 5-HT may remain longer in the extracellular space to continue neurotransmission. However, such argument does not support the observations that humans with depression have lower levels of 5-HT reuptake sites than healthy humans [122]. It might be that there is a mitigated 5-HT release and reduced levels of 5-HT in humans with depression to begin with, and a less 5-HT reuptake [107].

As we described, estrogens enhance 5-HT signaling via increasing 5-HT biosynthesis, upregulating expression and binding of receptors 5-HT2A and 5-HT2c, downregulating activity and expression of the 5-HT1A auto-receptor, decreasing expression of SERT gene and SERT protein allowing 5-HT to remain in the extracellular space for a longer period of time to continue neurotransmission, and decreasing 5-HT metabolism [107]. Consequently, the hypothesis of estrogen protection [123] claims that adjunctive estrogen treatment is beneficial at improving both symptoms of schizophrenia and the cognitive function, most notably in women. So far, the majority of studies on hormone replacement therapy for mood disorders have shown a positive response. Thus, estrogen has been demonstrated to improve mood in multiple mental illnesses, including major depressive disorder. Most recently, adjunctive estradiol treatment has been suggested as a promising treatment for women with comorbid depression and schizophrenia. In this direction, exploration of the impact of estrogen on serotonergic and other neurochemical pathways plus brain circuitry may guide not only the development of new hormone treatments but also assist in understanding the etiology of premenstrual dysphoric disorder, postnatal and perimenopausal depression, and even schizophrenia in women.

On the other hand, estrogens have shown that they do not always improve learning and memory. As an experimental example, acute administration of high doses of 17β-estradiol and progesterone can impair performance in the memory test of Morris water maze. And most importantly, there is coherence among human studies since high endogenous levels of 17β-estradiol are associated with poor performance on spatial tasks and cognitive function (Montreal Cognitive Assessment scale) and high dose of exogenous 17β-estradiol impairs recognition memory. It is fundamental to assume that estradiol exerts a curvilinear influence on hippocampal-dependent performance, with low and high levels impairing versus a medium dose improving performance on a variety of tasks [124]. Similar dose response has been observed in the rapid effects of estrogens on dendritic spines, therefore, studies on the effects of estrogens on cellular morphology should take dose response into account. Furthermore, long-term exposure to estrogens can similarly result in dose-dependent responses on learning and memory, with low levels of 17β-estradiol reinforcing spatial working memory and high levels of estradiol hampering spatial working and reference memory. Studies have also shown that, whereas there is a dose-dependent facilitation in contextual fear conditioning by 17β- and 17α-estradiol, estrone results in dose-dependent impairments in contextual fear conditioning. Thus, it is essential to consider that the dose, frequency of administrations, and type of estrogen(s) utilized along with the type of memory task performed and the time point estrogens are administered (during acquisition or retrieval), are critical to the learning outcomes [124].

10. Conclusion

This review has concentrated on some cellular processes and signaling pathways acting during homeostatic molecular remodeling and their potential involvement in the maladaptive plasticity occurring in multiple neuropathologic conditions such as neurodegeneration and neuropsychiatric disorders.

There seem to be independent mechanisms for regulating presynaptic and postsynaptic strength, and there is evidence for independent homeostatic mechanisms operating on global and local spatial scales.

Involvement of different pharmacological approaches to compensate neurotransmission imbalance are under study, which may be considered as potential therapeutic approaches in neuropathologic conditions.

Acknowledgements

This work was supported by the Extraordinary Chair "UCM Farmacia-CESIF" at the Universidad Complutense de Madrid, a collaboration agreement for organizing educational and scientific activities within the scope of competences of the Pharmacology and the Pharmaceutical Industry.

Conflict of interest

Nothing declared.

Author details

Sagrario Martin-Aragon*, Paloma Bermejo-Bescós, Pilar González and Juana Benedí
Department of Pharmacology, Pharmacognosy and Botany, School of Pharmacy, Complutense University, Madrid, Spain

*Address all correspondence to: smartina@ucm.es

IntechOpen

© 2019 The Author(s). Licensee IntechOpen. This chapter is distributed under the terms of the Creative Commons Attribution License (http://creativecommons.org/licenses/by/3.0), which permits unrestricted use, distribution, and reproduction in any medium, provided the original work is properly cited. (cc) BY

References

[1] Cheng A, Hou Y, Mattson MP. Mitochondria and neuroplasticity. ASN Neuro. 2010;2:e00045. DOI: 10.1042/AN20100019

[2] Todorova V, Blokland A. Mitochondria and synaptic plasticity in the mature and aging nervous system. Current Neuropharmacology. 2017;15: 166-173. DOI: 10.2174/1570159X14666160414111821

[3] Hanlon CD, Andrew DJ. Outside-in signaling—A brief review of GPCR signaling with a focus on the Drosophila GPCR family. Journal of Cell Science. 2015;128:3533-3542. DOI: 10.1242/jcs.175158

[4] Balua DT, Coyle JT. Neuroplasticity signaling pathways linked to the pathophysiology of schizophrenia. Neuroscience & Biobehavioral Reviews. 2011;35:848-870. DOI: 10.1016/j.neubiorev.2010.10.005

[5] Bosch M, Castro J, Saneyoshi T, Matsuno H, Sur M, Hayashi Y. Structural and molecular remodeling of dendritic spine substructures during long-term potentiation. Neuron. 2014; 82:444-459. DOI: 10.1016/j.neuron.2014.03.021

[6] Voglis G, Tavernarakis N. The role of synaptic ion channels in synaptic plasticity. EMBO Reports. 2006;7: 1104-1110. DOI: 10.1038/sj.embor.7400830

[7] Koponen E, Lakso M, Castrén E. Overexpression of the full-length neurotrophin receptor trkB regulates the expression of plasticity-related genes in mouse brain. Molecular Brain Research. 2004;130:81-94. DOI: 10.1016/j.molbrainres.2004.07.010

[8] Turrigiano GG. The self-tuning neuron: Synaptic scaling of excitatory synapses. Cell. 2008;135:422-435. DOI: 10.1016/j.cell.2008.10.008

[9] Lu B. BDNF and activity-dependent synaptic modulation. Learning & Memory. 2003;10:86-98. DOI: 10.1101/lm.54603

[10] Reimers JM, Loweth JA, Wolf ME. BDNF contributes to both rapid and homeostatic alterations in AMPA receptor surface expression in nucleus accumbens medium spiny neurons. European Journal of Neuroscience. 2014; 39:1159-1169. DOI: 10.1111/ejn.12422

[11] Skaper SD. Neurotrophic factors: An overview. Methods in Molecular Biology. 2018;1727:1-17. DOI: 10.1007/978-1-4939-7571-6_1

[12] Mitre M, Mariga A, Chao MV. Neurotrophin signalling: Novel insights into mechanisms and pathophysiology. Clinical Science (London). 2017;131: 13-23. DOI: 10.1042/CS20160044

[13] Du J, Feng L, Yang F, Lu B. Activity- and Ca(2+)-dependent modulation of surface expression of brain-derived neurotrophic factor receptors in hippocampal neurons. Journal of Cell Biology. 2000;150:1423-1434

[14] Castrén E, Pitkänen M, Sirviö J, Parsadanian A, Lindholm D, Thoenen H, et al. The induction of LTP increases BDNF and NGF mRNA but decreases NT-3 mRNA in the dentate gyrus. Neuroreport. 1993;4:895-898

[15] Kuipers SD, Trentani A, Tiron A, Mao X, Kuhl D, Bramham CR. BDNF-induced LTP is associated with rapid Arc/Arg3.1-dependent enhancement in adult hippocampal neurogenesis. Scientific Reports. 2016;6:21222. DOI: 10.1038/srep21222

[16] Mishchenko TA, Mitroshina EV, Usenko AV, Voronova NV,

Astrakhanova TA, Shirokova OM, et al. Features of neural network formation and their functions in primary hippocampal cultures in the context of chronic TrkB receptor system influence. Frontiers in Physiology. 2019;**9**:1925. DOI: 10.3389/fphys.2018.01925

[17] Markham A, Cameron I, Franklin P, Spedding M. BDNF increases rat brain mitochondrial respiratory coupling at complex I, but not complex II. European Journal of Neuroscience. 2004;**20**: 1189-1196. DOI: 10.1111/ j.1460-9568.2004.03578.x

[18] Katsu-Jiménez Y, Loría F, Corona JC, Díaz-Nido J. Gene transfer of brain-derived neurotrophic factor (BDNF) prevents neurodegeneration triggered by FXN deficiency. Molecular Therapy. 2016;**24**:877-889. DOI: 10.1038/ mt.2016.32

[19] Koh JY, Lim JS, Byun HR, Yoo MH. Abnormalities in the zinc-metalloprotease-BDNF axis may contribute to megalencephaly and cortical hyperconnectivity in young autism spectrum disorder patients. Molecular Brain. 2014;**7**:64. DOI: 10.1186/s13041-014-0064-z

[20] Yeo GS, Heisler LK. Unraveling the brain regulation of appetite: Lessons from genetics. Nature Neuroscience. 2012;**15**:1343-1349. DOI: 10.1038/ nn.3211

[21] Gray J, Yeo GS, Cox JJ, Morton J, Adlam AL, Keogh JM, et al. Hyperphagia, severe obesity, impaired cognitive function, and hyperactivity associated with functional loss of one copy of the brain-derived neurotrophic factor (BDNF) gene. Diabetes. 2006;**55**: 3366-3371. DOI: 10.2337/db06-0550

[22] Cunha RA. Adenosine: An endogenous regulator of the brain immune system. In: Lajtha A, Vizi ES, editors. Handbook of Neurochemistry and Molecular Neurobiology. New York: Springer Science; 2008. pp. 283-291. DOI: 10.1007/978-0-387-30398-7_12

[23] Fredholm BB, IJzerman AP, Jacobson KA, Linden J, Müller CE. Nomenclature and classification of adenosine receptors—An update. Pharmacological Reviews. 2011;**63**:1-34. DOI: 10.1124/pr.110.003285

[24] Pandolfo P, Machado NJ, Köfalvi A, Takahashi R, Cunha R. Caffeine regulates frontocorticostriatal dopamine transporter density and improves attention and cognitive deficits in an animal model of attention deficit hyperactivity disorder. European Neuropsychopharmacology. 2013;**23**: 317-328. DOI: 10.1016/j.euroneuro. 2012.04.011

[25] Sarantis K, Tsiamaki E, Kouvaros S, Papatheodoropoulos C, Angelatou F. Adenosine A_2A receptors permit mGluR5-evoked tyrosine phosphorylation of NR2B (Tyr1472) in rat hippocampus: A possible key mechanism in NMDA receptor modulation. Journal of Neurochemistry. 2015;**135**:714-726. DOI: 10.1111/ jnc.13291

[26] Rial D, Lemos C, Pinheiro H, Duarte JM, Gonçalves FQ, Real JI, et al. Depression as a glial-based synaptic dysfunction. Frontiers in Cellular Neuroscience. 2016;**9**:521. DOI: 10.3389/ fncel.2015.00521

[27] Cunha GM, Canas PM, Melo CS, Hockemeyer J, Müller CE, Oliveira CR, et al. Adenosine A2A receptor blockade prevents memory dysfunction caused by beta-amyloid peptides but not by scopolamine or MK-801. Experimental Neurology. 2008;**210**:776-781. DOI: 10.1016/j.expneurol.2007.11.013

[28] Costenla AR, Diógenes MJ, Canas PM, Rodrigues RJ, Nogueira C, Maroco J, et al. Enhanced role of adenosine A2A receptors in the modulation of LTP in the rat hippocampus upon ageing.

European Journal of Neuroscience. 2011;**34**:12-21. DOI: 10.1111/j.1460-9568.2011.07719.x

[29] Cunha RA, Vizi ES, Ribeiro JA, Sebastião AM. Preferential release of ATP and its extracellular catabolism as a source of adenosine upon high- but not low-frequency stimulation of rat hippocampal slices. Journal of Neurochemistry. 1996;**67**:2180-2187

[30] Viana da Silva S, Haberl MG, Zhang P, Bethge P, Lemos C, Gonçalves N, et al. Early synaptic deficits in the APP/PS1 mouse model of Alzheimer's disease involve neuronal adenosine A2A receptors. Nature Communications. 2016;**7**:11915. DOI: 10.1038/ncomms11915

[31] Chiodi V, Ferrante A, Ferraro L, Potenza RL, Armida M, Beggiato S, et al. Striatal denosine-cannabinoid receptor interactions in rats over-expressing adenosine A2A receptors. Journal of Neurochemistry. 2016;**136**:907-917. DOI: 10.1111/jnc.13421

[32] Chen J, Tan Z, Zeng L, Zhang X, He Y, Gao W, et al. Heterosynaptic long-term depression mediated by ATP released from astrocytes. Glia. 2013;**61**: 178-191. DOI: 10.1002/glia.22425

[33] Cunha RA. How does adenosine control neuronal dysfunction and neurodegeneration? Journal of Neurochemistry. 2016;**139**:1019-1055. DOI: 10.1111/jnc.13724

[34] Silva AC, Lemos C, Gonçalves FQ, Pliássova AV, Machado NJ, Silva HB, et al. Blockade of adenosine A2A receptors recovers early deficits of memory and plasticity in the triple transgenic mouse model of Alzheimer's disease. Neurobiology of Disease. 2018; **117**:72-81. DOI: 10.1016/j.nbd.2018.05.024

[35] Garthwaite J. From synaptically localized to volume transmission by nitric oxide. The Journal of Physiology. 2016;**594**:9-18. DOI: 10.1113/JP270297

[36] Szabadits E, Cserép C, Szonyi A, Fukazawa Y, Shigemoto R, Watanabe M, et al. NMDA receptors in hippocampal GABAergic synapses and their role in nitric oxide signaling. Journal of Neuroscience. 2011;**31**: 5893-5904. DOI: 10.1523/JNEUROSCI.5938-10.2011

[37] Wang JQ, Chu XP, Guo ML, Jin DZ, Xue B, Berry TJ, et al. Modulation of ionotropic glutamate receptors and acid-sensing ion channels by nitric oxide. Frontiers in Physiology. 2012;**3**: 164. DOI: 10.3389/fphys.2012.00164

[38] Shefa U, Kim D, Kim MS, Jeong NY, Jung J. Roles of gasotransmitters in synaptic plasticity and neuropsychiatric conditions. Neural Plasticity. 2018;**2018**: 1824713. DOI: 10.1155/2018/1824713

[39] Blasko J, Fabianova K, Martoncikova M, Sopkova D, Racekova E. Immunohistochemical evidence for the presence of synaptic connections of nitrergic neurons in the rat rostral migratory stream. Cellular and Molecular Neurobiology. 2013;**33**:753-757. DOI: 10.1007/s10571-013-9956-1

[40] Cooke RM, Mistry R, Challiss RA, Straub VA. Nitric oxide synthesis and cGMP production is important for neurite growth and synapse remodeling after axotomy. Journal of Neuroscience. 2013;**33**:5626-5637. DOI: 10.1523/JNEUROSCI.3659-12.2013

[41] Nisticò R, Cavallucci V, Piccinin S, Macrì S, Pignatelli M, Mehdawy B, et al. Insulin receptor β-subunit haploinsufficiency impairs hippocampal late-phase LTP and recognition memory. NeuroMolecular Medicine. 2012;**14**:262-269. DOI: 10.1007/s12017-012-8184-z

[42] Wilcock DM, Lewis MR, Van Nostrand WE, Davis J, Previti ML,

Gharkholonarehe N, et al. Progression of amyloid pathology to Alzheimer's disease pathology in an amyloid precursor protein transgenic mouse model by removal of nitric oxide synthase 2. Journal of Neuroscience. 2008;**28**:1537-1545. DOI: 10.1523/JNEUROSCI.5066-07.2008

[43] Chakroborty S, Stutzmann GE. Early calcium dysregulation in Alzheimer's disease: Setting the stage for synaptic dysfunction. Science China Life Sciences. 2011;**54**:752-762. DOI: 10.1007/s11427-011-4205-7

[44] Chakroborty S, Kim J, Schneider C, West AR, Stutzmann GE. Nitric oxide signaling is recruited as a compensatory mechanism for sustaining synaptic plasticity in Alzheimer's disease mice. Journal of Neuroscience. 2015;**35**: 6893-6902. DOI: 10.1523/JNEUROSCI.4002-14.2015

[45] Ratnayaka A, Marra V, Bush D, Burden JJ, Branco T, Staras K. Recruitment of resting vesicles into recycling pools supports NMDA receptor-dependent synaptic potentiation in cultured hippocampal neurons. The Journal of Physiology. 2012;**590**:1585-1597. DOI: 10.1113/jphysiol.2011.226688

[46] Zhao QF, Yu JT, Tan L. S-Nitrosylation in Alzheimer's disease. Molecular Neurobiology. 2015;**51**: 268-280. DOI: 10.1007/s12035-014-8672-2

[47] Zhihui Q. Modulating nitric oxide signaling in the CNS for Alzheimer's disease therapy. Future Medicinal Chemistry. 2013;**5**:1451-1468. DOI: 10.4155/fmc.13.111

[48] Padovan-Neto FE, Jurkowski L, Murray C, Stutzmann GE, Kwan M, Ghavami A, et al. Age- and sex-related changes in cortical and striatal nitric oxide synthase in the Q175 mouse model of Huntington's disease. Nitric Oxide. 2019;**83**:40-50. DOI: 10.1016/j.niox. 2018.12.002

[49] Garthwaite J. NO as a multimodal transmitter in the brain: Discovery and current status. British Journal of Pharmacology. 2019;**176**:197-211. DOI: 10.1111/bph.14532

[50] Wang B, Han S. Inhibition of Inducible Nitric Oxide Synthase Attenuates Deficits in Synaptic Plasticity and Brain Functions Following Traumatic Brain Injury. Cerebellum. 2018;**17**: 477-484. DOI: 10.1007/s12311-018-0934-5

[51] Liu Y, Zeng X, Hui Y, Zhu C, Wu J, Taylor DH, et al. Activation of α7 nicotinic acetylcholine receptors protects astrocytes against oxidative stress-induced apoptosis: Implications for Parkinson's disease. Neuropharmacology. 2015;**91**:87-96. DOI: 10.1016/j.neuropharm.2014. 11.028

[52] Sadigh-Eteghad S, Majdi A, Mahmoudi J, Golzari SE, Talebi M. Astrocytic and microglial nicotinic acetylcholine receptors: An overlooked issue in Alzheimer's disease. Journal of Neural Transmission (Vienna). 2016; **123**:1359-1367. DOI: 10.1007/s00702-016-1580-z

[53] Yu WF, Guan ZZ, Bogdanovic N, Nordberg A. High selective expression of alpha7 nicotinic receptors on astrocytes in the brains of patients with sporadic Alzheimer's disease and patients carrying Swedish APP 670/671 mutation: A possible association with neuritic plaques. Experimental Neurology. 2005;**192**:215-225. DOI: 10.1016/j.expneurol.2004.12.015

[54] Lee L, Kosuri P, Arancio O. Picomolar amyloid-beta peptides enhance spontaneous astrocyte calcium transients. Journal of Alzheimer's disease. 2014;**38**:49-62. DOI: 10.3233/JAD-130740

[55] Yakel JL. Nicotinic ACh receptors in the hippocampus: Role in excitability and plasticity. Nicotine & Tobacco Research. 2012;**14**:1249-1257. DOI: 10.1093/ntr/nts091

[56] Pirttimaki TM, Codadu NK, Awni A, Pratik P, Nagel DA, Hill EJ, et al. α7 nicotinic receptor-mediated astrocytic gliotransmitter release: Aβ effects in a preclinical Alzheimer's mouse model. PLoS One. 2013;**8**:e81828. DOI: 10.1371/journal.pone.0081828

[57] Beggiato S, Antonelli T, Tomasini MC, Tanganelli S, Fuxe K, Schwarcz R, et al. Kynurenic acid, by targeting alpha7 nicotinic acetylcholine receptors, modulates extracellular GABA levels in the rat striatum in vivo. European Journal of Neuroscience. 2013;**37**: 1470-1477. DOI: 10.1111/ejn.12160

[58] Liu Y, Hu J, Wu J, Zhu C, Hui Y, Han Y, et al. α7 nicotinic acetylcholine receptor-mediated neuroprotection against dopaminergic neuron loss in an MPTP mouse model via inhibition of astrocyte activation. Journal of Neuroinflammation. 2012;**9**:2094-2099. DOI: 10.1186/1742-2094-9-98

[59] Takarada T, Nakamichi N, Kawagoe H, Ogura M, Fukumori R, Nakazato R, et al. Possible neuroprotective property of nicotinic acetylcholine receptors in association with predominant upregulation of glial cell line-derived neurotrophic factor in astrocytes. Journal of Neuroscience Research. 2012;**90**:2074-2085. DOI: 10.1002/jnr.23101. E

[60] Konishi Y, Yang L-B, He P, Lindholm K, Lu B, Li R, et al. Deficiency of GDNF receptor GFRα1 in Alzheimer's neurons results in neuronal death. Journal of Neuroscience Research. 2014; **34**:13127-13138. DOI: 10.1523/JNEUROSCI.2582-13.2014

[61] Metna-Laurent M, Marsicano G. Rising stars: Modulation of brain functions by astroglial type-1 cannabinoid receptors. Glia. 2015;**63**: 353-364. DOI: 10.1002/glia.22773

[62] Devane WA, Hanus L, Breuer A, Pertwee RG, Stevenson LA, Griffin G, et al. Isolation and structure of a brain constituent that binds to the cannabinoid receptor. Science. 1992;**258**: 1946-1949

[63] Han J, Kesner P, Metna-Laurent M, Duan T, Xu L, Georges F, et al. Acute cannabinoids impair working memory through astroglial CB1 receptor modulation of hippocampal LTD. Cell. 2012;**148**:1039-1050. DOI: 10.1016/j.cell.2012.01.037

[64] Loría F, Petrosino S, Hernangómez M, Mestre L, Spagnolo A, Correa F, et al. An endocannabinoid tone limits excitotoxicity in vitro and in a model of multiple sclerosis. Neurobiology of Disease. 2010;**37**:166-176. DOI: 10.1016/j.nbd.2009.09.020

[65] Navarrete M, Araque A. Endocannabinoids mediate neuron-astrocyte communication. Neuron. 2008;**57**:883-893. DOI: 10.1016/j.neuron.2008.01.029

[66] Navarrete M, Diez A, Araque A. Astrocytes in endocannabinoid signalling. Philosophical Transactions of the Royal Society B: Biological Sciences. 2014;**369**:20130599-20130599. DOI: 10.1098/rstb.2013.0599

[67] Soria-Gómez E, Massa F, Bellocchio L, Rueda-Orozco PE, Ciofi P, Cota D, et al. Cannabinoid type-1 receptors in the paraventricular nucleus of the hypothalamus inhibit stimulated food intake. Neuroscience. 2014;**263**:46-53. DOI: 10.1016/j.neuroscience.2014.01.005

[68] Bakota L, Ussif A, Jeserich G, Brandt R. Systemic and network functions of the microtubule-associated protein tau: Implications for tau-based therapies. Molecular and Cellular

Neuroscience. 2017;**84**:132-141. DOI: 10.1016/j.mcn.2017.03.003

[69] Penazzi L, Bakota L, Brandt R. Microtubule dynamics in neuronal development, plasticity, and neurodegeneration. International Review of Cell and Molecular Biology. 2016;**321**:89-169. DOI: 10.1016/bs.ircmb.2015.09.004

[70] Arendt T, Stieler JT, Holzer M. Tau and tauopathies. Brain Research Bulletin. 2016;**126**:238-292. DOI: 10.1016/j.brainresbull.2016.08.018

[71] Uversky VN. Intrinsically disordered proteins and their (disordered) proteomes in neurodegenerative disorders. Frontiers in Aging Neuroscience. 2015;**7**:18. DOI: 10.3389/fnagi.2015.00018

[72] Cantero L, Moreno-Lopez B, Portillo F, Rubio A, Hita-Yanez E, Avila J. Role of tau protein on neocortical and hippocampal oscillatory patterns. Hippocampus. 2011;**21**:827-834. DOI: 10.1002/hipo.20798

[73] Regan P, Piers T, Yi JH, Kim DH, Huh S, Park SJ, et al. Tau phosphorylation at serine 396 residue is required for hippocampal LTD. Journal of Neuroscience. 2015;**35**:4804-4812. DOI: 10.1523/JNEUROSCI.2842-14.2015

[74] Pooler AM, Phillips EC, Lau DH, Noble W, Hanger DP. Physiological release of endogenous tau is stimulated by neuronal activity. EMBO Reports. 2013;**14**:389-394. DOI: 10.1038/embor.2013.15

[75] Plouffe V, Mohamed NV, Rivest-McGraw J, Bertrand J, Lauzon M, Leclerc N. Hyperphosphorylation and cleavage at D421 enhance tau secretion. PLoS One. 2012;**7**:e36873. DOI: 10.1371/journal.pone.0036873

[76] Goedert M. Neurodegeneration. Alzheimer's and Parkinson's diseases:

the prion concept in relation to assembled Abeta, tau, and alpha-synuclein. Science. 2015;**349**(6248): 1255555. DOI: 10.1126/science.1255555

[77] Fá M, Puzzo D, Piacentini R, Staniszewski A, Zhang H, Baltrons MA, et al. Extracellular Tau oligomers produce an immediate impairment of LTP and memory. Scientific Reports. 2016;**6**:19393. DOI: 10.1038/srep19393

[78] Bullmann T, Seeger G, Stieler J, Hanics J, Reimann K, Kretzschmann TP, et al. Tau phosphorylation-associated spine regression does not impair hippocampal-dependent memory in hibernating golden hamsters. Hippocampus. 2016;**26**:301-318. DOI: 10.1002/hipo.22522

[79] Siano G, Varisco M, Caiazza MC, Quercioli V, Mainardi M, Ippolito C, et al. Tau modulates VGluT1 expression. Journal of Molecular Biology. 2019;**431**: 873-884. DOI: 10.1016/j.jmb.2019.01.023

[80] Miki T, Yokota O, Takenoshita S, Mori Y, Yamazaki K, Ozaki Y, et al. Frontotemporal lobar degeneration due to P301L tau mutation showing apathy and severe frontal atrophy but lacking other behavioral changes: A case report and literature review. Neuropathology. 2018; **38**:268-280. DOI: 10.1111/neup.12441

[81] Nusse R, Clevers H. Wnt/β-catenin Signaling, disease, and emerging therapeutic modalities. Cell. 2017;**169**: 985-999. DOI: 10.1016/j.cell.2017.05.016

[82] Oliva CA, Montecinos-Oliva C, Inestrosa NC. Wnt Signaling in the central nervous system: New insights in health and disease. Progress in Molecular Biology and Translational Science. 2018;**153**:81-130. DOI: 10.1016/bs.pmbts.2017.11.018

[83] Speese SD, Budnik V. Wnts: Up-and-coming at the synapse. Trends

in Neurosciences. 2007;**30**:268-275. DOI: 10.1016/j.tins.2007.04.003

[84] McLeod F, Salinas PC. Wnt proteins as modulators of synaptic plasticity. Current Opinion in Neurobiology. 2018; **53**:90-95. DOI: 10.1016/j.conb.2018.06.003

[85] Ciani L, Boyle KA, Dickins E, Sahores M, Anane D, Lopes DM, et al. Wnt7a signaling promotes dendritic spine growth and synaptic strength through Ca(2)(+)/calmodulin-dependent protein kinase II. Proceedings of the National Academy of Sciences of the USA. 2011;**108**: 10732-10737. DOI: 10.1073/pnas.1018132108

[86] Cuitino L, Godoy JA, Farias GG, Couve A, Bonansco C, Fuenzalida M, et al. Wnt-5a modulates recycling of functional GABAA receptors on hippocampal neurons. Journal of Neuroscience. 2010;**30**:8411-8420. DOI: 10.1523/JNEUROSCI.5736-09.2010

[87] Sahores M, Gibb A, Salinas PC. Frizzled-5, a receptor for the synaptic organizer Wnt7a, regulates activity-mediated synaptogenesis. Development. 2010;**137**:2215-2225. DOI: 10.1242/dev.046722

[88] McLeod F, Bossio A, Marzo A, Ciani L, Sibilla S, Hannan S, et al. Wnt signaling mediates LTP-dependent spine plasticity and AMPAR localization through Frizzled-7 receptors. Cell Reports. 2018;**23**:1-12. DOI: 10.1016/j.celrep.2018.03.119

[89] Cerpa W, Gambrill A, Inestrosa NC, Barria A. Regulation of NMDA-receptor synaptic transmission by Wnt signaling. Journal of Neuroscience. 2011;**31**: 9466-9471. DOI: 10.1523/JNEUROSCI.6311-10.2011

[90] Galli S, Lopes DM, Ammari R, Kopra J, Millar SE, Gibb A, et al.

Deficient Wnt signalling triggers striatal synaptic degeneration and impaired motor behaviour in adult mice. Nature Communications. 2014;**5**:4992. DOI: 10.1038/ncomms5992

[91] Marzo A, Galli S, Lopes D, McLeod F, Podpolny M, Segovia-Roldan M, et al. Reversal of synapse degeneration by restoring Wnt signaling in the adult hippocampus. Current Biology. 2016;**26**: 2551-2561. DOI: 10.1016/j.cub.2016.07.024

[92] Purro SA, Dickins EM, Salinas PC. The secreted Wnt antagonist Dickkopf-1 is required for amyloid beta-mediated synaptic loss. Journal of Neuroscience. 2012;**32**:3492-3498. DOI: 10.1523/JNEUROSCI.4562-11.2012

[93] De Ferrari GV, Papassotiropoulos A, Biechele T, Wavrant De-Vrieze F, Avila ME, Major MB, et al. Common genetic variation within the low-density lipoprotein receptor-related protein 6 and late-onset Alzheimer's disease. Proceedings of the National Academy of Sciences of the USA. 2007;**104**:9434-9439. DOI: 10.1073/pnas.0603523104

[94] Liu CC, Tsai CW, Deak F, Rogers J, Penuliar M, Sung YM, et al. Deficiency in LRP6-mediated Wnt signaling contributes to synaptic abnormalities and amyloid pathology in Alzheimer's disease. Neuron. 2014;**84**:63-77. DOI: 10.1016/j.neuron.2014.08.048

[95] Holm MM, Kaiser J, Schwab ME. Extracellular vesicles: Multimodal envoys in neural maintenance and repair. Trends in Neurosciences. 2018;**41**:360-372. DOI: 10.1016/j.tins.2018.03.006

[96] Riganti L, Antonucci F, Gabrielli M, Prada I, Giussani P, Viani P, et al. Sphingosine-1-phosphate (S1P) impacts presynaptic functions by regulating synapsini localization in the presynaptic compartment. Journal of Neuroscience. 2016;**36**:4624-4634. DOI: 10.1523/JNEUROSCI.3588-15.2016

[97] Thompson AG, Gray E, Heman-Ackah SM, Mäger I, Talbot K, Andaloussi SE, et al. Extracellular vesicles in neurodegenerative disease—Pathogenesis to biomarkers. Nature Reviews Neurology. 2016;**12**:346-357. DOI: 10.1038/nrneurol.2016.68

[98] Kumar A, Stoica BA, Loane DJ, Yang M, Abulwerdi G, Khan N, et al. Microglial-derived microparticles mediate neuroinflammation after traumatic brain injury. Journal of Neuroinflammation. 2017;**14**:47. DOI: 10.1186/s12974-017-0819-4

[99] Chivet M, Javalet C, Hemming F, Pernet-Gallay K, Laulagnier K, Fraboulet S, et al. Exosomes as a novel way of interneuronal communication. Biochemical Society Transactions. 2013;**41**:241-244. DOI: 10.1042/BST20120266

[100] Korkut C, Ataman B, Ramachandran P, Ashley J, Barria R, Gherbesi N, et al. Trans-synaptic transmission of vesicular Wnt signals through Evi/Wntless. Cell. 2009;**139**: 393-404. DOI: 10.1016/j.cell.2009.07.051

[101] Pastuzyn ED, Day CE, Kearns RB, Kyrke-Smith M, Taibi AV, McCormick J, et al. The neuronal gene Arc encodes a repurposed retrotransposon Gag protein that mediates intercellular RNA transfer. 2018;**172**(1–2):275-288.e18. DOI: 10.1016/j.cell.2017.12.024

[102] Ashley J, Cordy B, Lucia D, Fradkin LG, Budnik V, Thomson T. Retrovirus-like gag protein Arc1 binds RNA and traffics across synaptic boutons. Cell. 2018;**172**:262-274.e11. DOI: 10.1016/j.cell.2017.12.022

[103] Morel L, Regan M, Higashimori H, Ng SK, Esau C, Vidensky S, et al. Neuronal exosomal miRNA-dependent translational regulation of astroglial glutamate transporter GLT1. Journal of Biological Chemistry. 2013;**288**: 7105-7116. DOI: 10.1074/jbc. M112.410944

[104] Frühbeis C, Fröhlich D, Kuo WP, Amphornrat J, Thilemann S, Saab AS, et al. Neurotransmitter-triggered transfer of exosomes mediates oligodendrocyte-neuron communication. PLoS Biology. 2013;**11**: e1001604. DOI: 10.1371/journal. pbio.1001604

[105] Antonucci F, Turola E, Riganti L, Caleo M, Gabrielli M, Perrotta C, et al. Microvesicles released from microglia stimulate synaptic activity via enhanced sphingolipid metabolism. The EMBO Journal. 2012;**31**:1231-1240. DOI: 10.1038/emboj.2011.489

[106] Laso-García F, Ramos-Cejudo J, Carrillo-Salinas FJ, Otero-Ortega L, Feliú A, Gómez-de Frutos M, et al. Therapeutic potential of extracellular vesicles derived from human mesenchymal stem cells in a model of progressive multiple sclerosis. PLoS One. 2018;**13**:e0202590. DOI: 10.1371/ journal.pone.0202590

[107] Krolick KN, Zhu Q, Shi H. Effects of estrogens on central nervous system neurotransmission: Implications for sex differences in mental disorders. Progress in Molecular Biology and Translational Science. 2018;**160**:105-171. DOI: 10.1016/bs.pmbts.2018.07.008

[108] Greenberg GD, Trainor BC. Sex differences in the social behavior network and mesolimbic dopamine system. In: Shansky RM, editor. Sex Differences in the Central Nervous System. San Diego: Academic Press; 2016. pp. 77-106. DOI: 10.1016/B978-0-12-802114-9.00004-4

[109] Becker JB. Sexual differentiation of motivation: A novel mechanism? Hormones and Behavior. 2009;**55**: 646-654. DOI: 10.1016/j. yhbeh.2009.03.014

[110] Pecins-Thompson M, Brown NA, Kohama SG, Bethea CL. Ovarian steroid regulation of tryptophan hydroxylase

mRNA expression in rhesus macaques. Journal of Neuroscience. 1996;**16**: 7021-7029

[111] Lu NZ, Shlaes TA, Gundlah C, Dziennis SE, Lyle RE, Bethea CL. Ovarian steroid action on tryptophan hydroxylase protein and serotonin compared to localization of ovarian steroid receptors in midbrain of Guinea pigs. Endocrine. 1999;**11**:257-267. DOI: 10.1385/ENDO:11:3:257

[112] Kuhn DM, Arthur R, States JC. Phosphorylation and activation of brain tryptophan hydroxylase: Identification of serine-58 as a substrate site for protein kinase A. Journal of Neurochemistry. 1997;**68**:2220-2223

[113] Sumner BEH, Fink G. Testosterone as well as estrogen increases serotonin2A receptor mRNA and binding site densities in the male rat brain. Molecular Brain Research. 1998;**59**:205-214

[114] Burnet PWJ, Eastwood SL, Lacey K, Harrison PJ. The distribution of 5-HT1A and 5-HT2A receptor mRNA in human brain. Brain Research. 1995;**676**:157-168

[115] Biver F, Lotstra F, Monclus M, Wikler D, Damhaut P, Mendlewicz J, et al. Sex difference in 5HT2 receptor in the living human brain. Neuroscience Letters. 1996;**204**:25-28

[116] Sumner BEH, Fink G. Estrogen increases the density of 5-hydroxytryptamine (2A) receptors in cerebral cortex and nucleus accumbens in the female rat. The Journal of Steroid Biochemistry and Molecular Biology. 1995;**54**:15-20

[117] Cyr M, Bossé R, Di Paolo T. Gonadal hormones modulate 5-hydroxytryptamine 2A receptors: Emphasis on the rat frontal cortex. Neuroscience. 1998;**83**:829-836

[118] Gundlah C, Pecins-Thompson M, Schutzer WE, Bethea CL. Ovarian

steroid effects on serotonin 1A, 2A and 2C receptor mRNA in macaque hypothalamus. Molecular Brain Research. 1999;**63**:325-339

[119] Bohmaker K, Eison AS, Yocca FD, Meller E. Comparative effects of chronic 8-OH-DPAT, gepirone and ipsapirone treatment on the sensitivity of somatodendritic 5-HT1A autoreceptors. Neuropharmacology. 1993;**32**:527-534

[120] Raymond JR, Mukhin YV, Gettys TW, Garnovskaya MN. The recombinant 5-HT1A receptor: G protein coupling and signalling pathways. British Journal of Pharmacology. 1999;**127**:1751-1764. DOI: 10.1038/sj.bjp.0702723

[121] Hoffman BJ, Hansson SR, Mezey E, Palkovits M. Localization and dynamic regulation of biogenic amine transporters in the mammalian central nervous system. Frontiers in Neuroendocrinology. 1998;**19**:187-231. DOI: 10.1006/frne.1998.0168

[122] Malison RT, Price LH, Berman R, van Dyck CH, Pelton GH, Carpenter L, et al. Reduced brain serotonin transporter availability in major depression as measured by [123I]-2β-carbomethoxy-3β-(4-iodophenyl) tropane and single photon emission computed tomography. Biological Psychiatry. 1998;**44**:1090-1098

[123] Lascurain MB, Camuñas-Palacín A, Thomas N, Breadon C, Gavrilidis E, Hudaib AR, et al. Improvement in depression with oestrogen treatment in women with schizophrenia. Archives of Women's Mental Health. 2019 Mar 21. DOI: 10.1007/s00737-019-00959-3. [Epub ahead of print]

[124] Sheppard PAS, Choleris E, Galea LAM. Structural plasticity of the hippocampus in response to estrogens in female rodents. Molecular Brain. 2019; **12**:22. DOI: 10.1186/s13041-019-0442-7

Chapter 4

The Pharmacological Effects of Herbs on Catecholamine Signaling

Nobuyuki Yanagihara, Xiaoja Li, Yumiko Toyohira,
Noriaki Satoh, Hui Shao, Yasuhiro Nozaki, Shin Ishikane,
Fumi Takahashi, Ryo Okada, Hideyuki Kobayashi,
Masato Tsutsui and Taizo Kita

Abstract

Herbs have many biologically and pharmacologically active compounds such as flavonoids and stilbenes. They have been used in remedies for various disorders. Here we review the effects of herbs on catecholamine synthesis and secretion in cultured bovine adrenal medullary cells. Ikarisoside A (1.0–100 μM), a flavonol glycoside, inhibited the catecholamine secretion induced by acetylcholine (0.3 mM). This inhibition was associated with the suppression of $^{22}Na^+$ and $^{45}Ca^{2+}$ influx induced by acetylcholine. The ethanol extract (0.0003–0.005%) of matsufushi (extract of pine nodules) inhibited the catecholamine secretion induced by acetylcholine. SJ-2, one of the stilbene compounds isolated from matsufushi, inhibited acetylcholine-induced catecholamine secretion. Matsufushi extract and SJ-2 reversibly inhibited acetylcholine-induced Na^+ currents in *Xenopus* oocytes expressed with α3β4nicotinic acetylcholine receptors. Sweet tea is the processed leaves of *Hydrangea macrophylla*. The extract of sweet tea (0.3–1.0 mg/ml) suppressed catecholamine secretion induced by acetylcholine (0.3 mM). Moreover, sweet tea (0.1–1.0 mg/ml), ikarisoside A (1.0–100 μM), and matsufushi (0.001–0.003%) or SJ-2 (10–30 μM) inhibited acetylcholine-induced ^{14}C-catecholamine synthesis from ^{14}C-tyrosine. These findings indicate that ikarisoside A, matsufushi (or SJ-2), and sweet tea inhibit the catecholamine secretion and synthesis induced by acetylcholine in cultured bovine adrenal medullary cells and probably in sympathetic neurons.

Keywords: adrenal medullary cells, catecholamine secretion, ikarisoside A, matsufushi, sweet tea

1. Introduction

Since herbs have many biologically and pharmacologically active compounds such as flavonoids and stilbenes, they have been used in remedies for various disorders. A high dietary intake of herbs has become a focus of research because of herbs' potential to reduce the risks of diseases such as hypertension, coronary heart disease, diabetes, and cancers [1, 2]. Flavonoids are a group of plant secondary metabolites with variable phenolic structures, and they are found in plants, fruits, vegetables, roots, stems, flowers, wine, and tea [3, 4]. Over 5000 individual flavonoids have been reported [5], and 6 principal groups of flavonoids

IntechOpen

(flavones, flavonols, flavanones, flavanols, isoflavones, and anthocyanidins) are relatively common in human diets [1]. Polyphenol stilbenes have attracted scientific attention. For example, resveratrol (*trans*-3,4′,5-trihydroxy- stilbene) is a natural phytoestrogen found in grapes, berries, and red wine [6, 7] that was reported to be implicated in the beneficial effect of red wine, i.e., the lower incidence of coronary artery disease in certain populations such as the French and the Greeks, despite diets rich in saturated fat and a rate of high smoking, which has been dubbed the "French paradox" [8].

In the human body, the most abundant catecholamines are adrenaline, nor-adrenaline, and dopamine, all of which are produced from phenylalanine and/or tyrosine. Catecholamines are biosynthesized mainly in the adrenal medulla, the postganglionic fibers of the sympathetic nervous system, and the central nervous system [2, 9, 10]. Catecholamines play very important roles in aspects of the cardio-vascular system such as heart rate and blood pressure, blood glucose levels, and the general functions of the central and peripheral sympathetic nervous system [9].

Adrenal medullary cells derived from embryonic neural crests are functionally homologous to sympathetic postganglionic neurons [2, 10]. Our research demonstrated that in cultured bovine adrenal medullary cells, at least three distinct types of ionic channels participate in catecholamine secretion, including nicotinic acetylcholine receptor (nAChR)-ion channels, voltage-dependent Na^+ channels, and voltage-dependent Ca^{2+} channels [2, 11]. In these cells, the Na^+ influx induced by acetylcholine (ACh) via nAChR-ion channels or by veratridine via voltage-dependent Na^+ channels is a prerequisite for Ca^{2+} influx via the activation of voltage-dependent Ca^{2+} channels and subsequent catecholamine secretion; in contrast, high K^+ directly gates voltage-dependent Ca^{2+} channels to increase the Ca^{2+} influx without increasing the $^{22}Na^+$ influx [10, 11] (**Figure 1**). ACh-induced Ca^{2+} influx is also a prerequisite for the stimulation of catecholamine synthesis associated with the activation of tyrosine hydroxylase [2, 12–15]. The mechanisms underlying the stimulation of catecholamine synthesis and secretion mediated by these ion channels in adrenal medullary cells are thought to be similar to those of

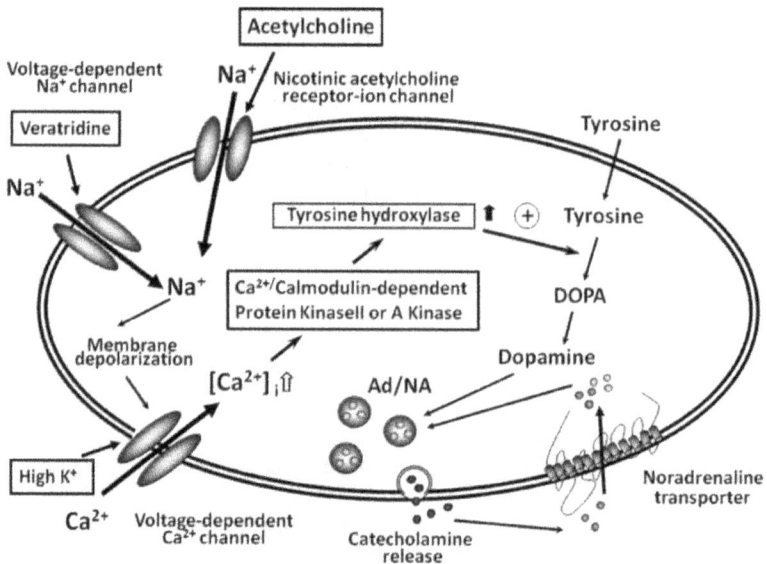

Figure 1.
The mechanism underlying the regulation of catecholamine synthesis, secretion, and reuptake in bovine adrenal medullary cells.

noradrenaline in the sympathetic neurons and brain noradrenergic neurons [2]. Thus, adrenal medullary cells have provided a good model for the detailed analysis of antipsychotic [16], cardiovascular [17], and analgesic [18] drugs that act on catecholamine synthesis, secretion, and reuptake [2].

We have demonstrated the effects of several flavonoids and polyphenol stilbenes on catecholamine synthesis and secretion. For example, the treatment of bovine adrenal medullary cells with daidzein (an isoflavone derived from soy beans) stimulated basal catecholamine synthesis but inhibited the catecholamine synthesis and secretion induced by ACh [2, 19]. Genistein (another isoflavone in soy beans) but not daidzein stimulated the function of noradrenaline transporter in a human neuroblastoma cell line, SK-N-SH cells [2, 20]. Nobiletin (a compound of polyme-thoxy flavone in citrus fruits) stimulated the basal synthesis and secretion of cat-echolamines, but it suppressed both the ACh-induced synthesis of catecholamines and ACh-induced secretion of catecholamines [2, 21]. Resveratrol also inhibited the catecholamine synthesis and secretion induced by ACh [2, 22].

The present review summarizes our recent and current studies of the phar-macological effects of herbs and their components, i.e., ikarisoside A (a flavonol glycoside); matsufushi (extract of pine nodules), one of matsufushi's stilbene components (SJ-2); and sweet tea on the catecholamine signaling induced by ACh in cultured bovine adrenal medullary cells and on ACh-induced Na^+ current in *Xenopus* oocytes expressing $\alpha3\beta4$ nAChRs.

2. Inhibitory effects of ikarisoside A, but not its aglycon, on the catecholamine secretion and synthesis induced by ACh

Ikarisoside A is a natural flavonol glycoside derived from plants of the genus *Epimedium*, which have been used in traditional Chinese medicine as tonics, antirheumatics, and aphrodisiacs [10, 23, 24], and is used as a tonic supplement in Japan. Ikarisoside A has antioxidant and anti-inflammatory effects [23] and anti-osteoporosis effects [10, 25]. Icariin, another flavonoid in the genus *Epimedium*, has an anti-stress effect in the forced swimming test in mice [26].

We observed that ikarisoside A (1–100 μM) concentration dependently inhibited the secretion of catecholamines induced by ACh (0.3 m) (**Figure 2A**), but not the secretion of catecholamines induced by veratridine and 56 mK⁺ [10]. Ikarisoside A also suppressed the $^{22}Na^+$ influx and $^{45}Ca^{2+}$ influx induced by ACh in a concentration-dependent manner similar to that of catecholamine secretion (**Figure 2B, C**) [10]. Ikarisoside A is a flavonol glycoside with one rhamnose at the 3 position in the chemi-cal structure. The aglycon of ikarisoside A is 3,5,7-trihydroxy-2-(4-hydroxyphenyl)-8-(3-methylbut-2-enyl)-4*H*-chromen-4one (**Figure 3A**).
It is interesting to note that the aglycon of ikarisoside A had little effect on catechol-amine secretion induced by ACh (0.3 m) (**Figure 3B**), suggesting that the rhamnose moiety at the 3 position of ikarisoside A is essential to inhibit the function of nAChR-ion channels [10]. Ikarisoside A (1.0–100 or 10–100 μM) inhibited ACh (0.3 mM)-induced ^{14}C-catecholamine synthesis from ^{14}C-tyrosine and tyrosine hydroxylase activity [10].

3. Inhibitory effects of matsufushi and its stilbene component, SJ-2, on the catecholamine synthesis and secretion induced by ACh

Pine nodules of *Pinus tabulaeformis* or *Pinus massoniana* are formed by pine bark proliferation at places on the trunk or limbs that have undergone damage, either

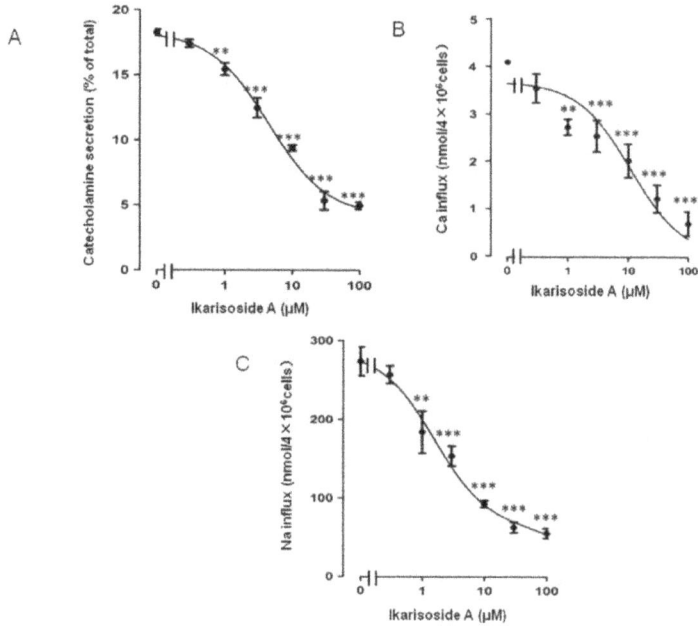

Figure 2.
Effects of ikarisoside A on ACh-induced catecholamine secretion (A), $^{45}Ca^{2+}$ influx (B), and $^{22}Na^+$ influx (C). (A) Cultured bovine adrenal medullary cells (10^6/well) were stimulated with ACh (300 μM) in the presence or absence of ikarisoside A (0.3–100 μM) for 10 min at 37°C. Catecholamine secretion is expressed as a percentage of the total catecholamines in the cells. (B and C) Cells (4 × 10^6/well) are stimulated with ACh (300 μM) and 1.5 μCi of $^{45}CaCl_2$ (B) or $^{22}NaCl$ (C) in the presence or absence of ikarisoside A (0.3–100 μM) for 5 min at 37°C. $^{45}Ca^{2+}$ influx and $^{22}Na^+$ influx were expressed as nmol/4 × 10^6 cells. Data are means ± SEM from three separate experiments carried out in triplicate. $^{**}P < 0.01$ and $^{***}P < 0.001$ vs. ACh alone (by one-way ANOVA with Dunnett's multiple comparison post hoc test) (cited from [25]).

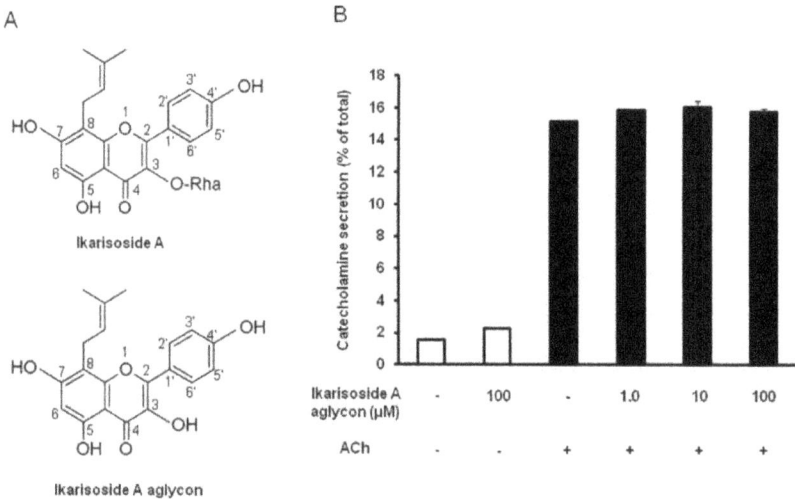

Figure 3.
Structures of ikarisoside A and its aglycon (A) and the effect of aglycon of ikarisoside A on the catecholamine secretion induced by ACh (0.3 mM) (B). (A) Chemical structures of ikarisoside A and its aglycon (3,5,7-trihydroxy-2-(4-hydroxyphenyl)-8- (3-methylbut-2-enyl)-4H-chromen-4-one). (B) Cells (10^6/well) were incubated with or without aglycon of ikarisoside A (1–100 μM) and ACh (300 μM) for 10 min at 37°C. Catecholamine secretion is expressed as a percentage of the total. Data are means ± SEM from three separate experiments carried out in triplicate (cited from [25]).

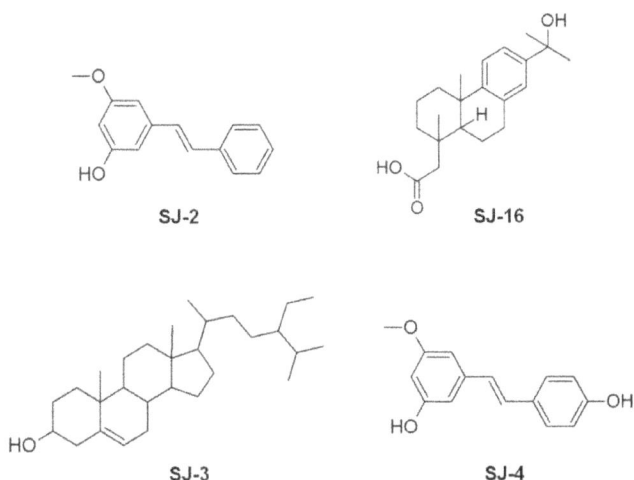

Figure 4.
Chemical structures of SJ-2, SJ-3, SJ-4, and SJ-16 (cited from [28]).

by pests or physical injury [27]. The effective curative components in pine nodule extract (matsufushi) have been used as an analgesic for joint pain, rheumatism, neuralgia, dysmenorrhea, and other complaints in traditional Chinese medicine [27–29]. Matsufushi is used as a healthy supplement in Japan.

Matsufushi ethanol extract (0.0003–0.005%) concentration dependently inhibited the catecholamine secretion and $^{45}Ca^{2+}$ influx induced by ACh (0.3 mM) and veratridine (0.1 mM), but not 56 mM K$^+$ in cultured bovine adrenal medullary cells [27]. Four compounds (SJ-2, SL-3, SJ-4, and SJ-16) were isolated from matsufushi extract (**Figure 4**). SJ-2, a phenol stilbene, and the mixture of four compounds (Mix4; SJ-2, SJ-3, SJ-4, and SJ-16), but not each of the other separate compounds, inhibited the catecholamine secretion (**Figure 5**) and $^{45}Ca^{2+}$ influx [27] induced by ACh (0.3 mM). In *Xenopus* oocytes

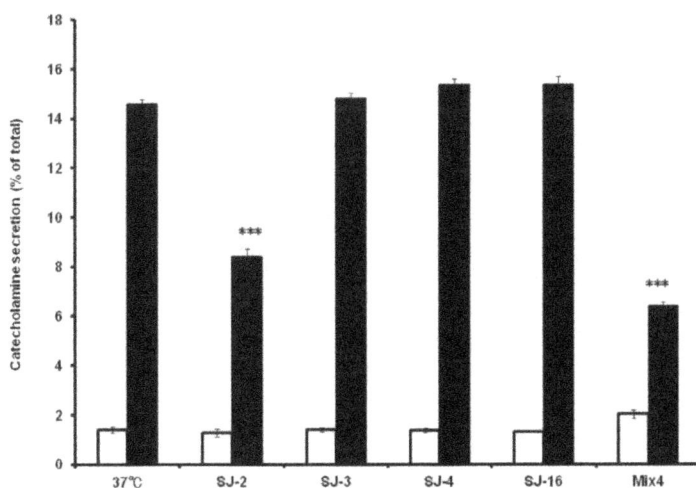

Figure 5.
*Effects of SJ-2, SJ-3, SJ-4, SJ-16, and their mixture (Mix4) on catecholamine secretion induced by ACh in cultured bovine adrenal medullary cells. The cells (10^6/well) were incubated with or without SJ-2 (10 μM), SJ-3 (10 μM), SJ-4 (10 μM), C-16 (10 μM), and their mixture (Mix 4) (10 μM) for 10 min at 37°C. Catecholamine secretion is expressed as a percentage of the total catecholamines in the cells. Data are means ± SEM from three separate experiments carried out in triplicate. ***$P < 0.001$ vs. ACh alone. Rha: rhamnose (cited from [28]).*

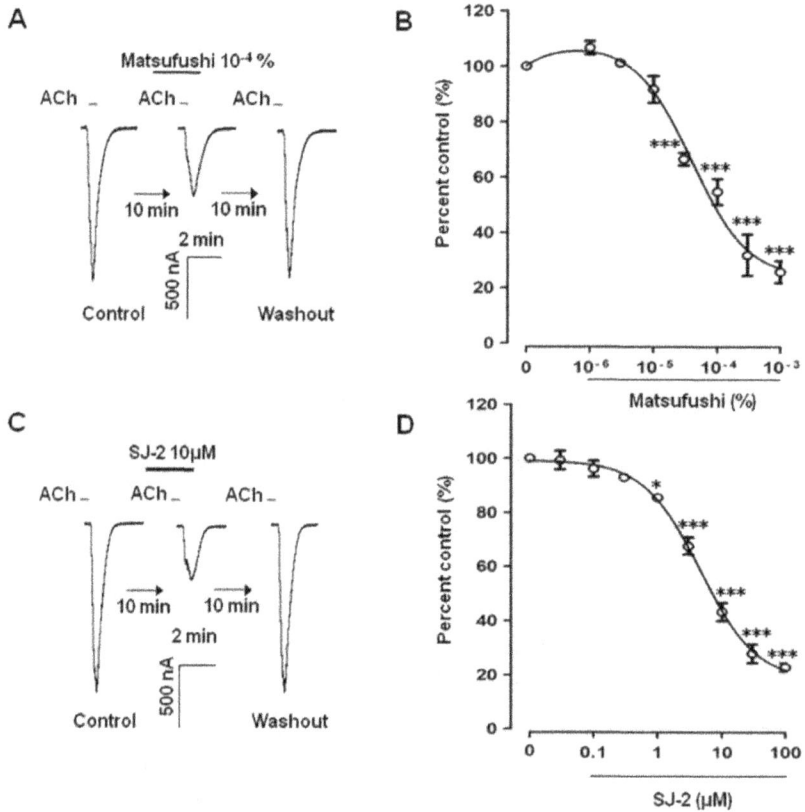

Figure 6.
*Effects of ethanol extract of matsufushi and SJ-2 on inward currents induced by ACh in Xenopus oocytes expressing rat α3β4 nAChRs. Representative traces from a single Xenopus oocyte are shown. The currents of matsufushi-treated (**A**) and SJ-2-treated (**C**) oocytes were recorded for 10 min after recording of the control currents, and the washout currents were obtained for 10 min after matsufushi extract and SJ-2 treatment. Matsufushi extract (0.0001%) and SJ-2 (10 μM) suppressed the currents induced by the EC50 (0.2 mM) of ACh, and the inhibitory effects were reversible. Concentration-response curve for the inhibitory effects of matsufushi extract (**B**) and SJ-2 (**D**) on ACh-induced currents. The peak current amplitude in the presence of matsufushi extract and SJ-2 was normalized to that of the control, and the effects are expressed as percentages of the control. Data are presented as means ± SEM from four separate experiments carried out in triplicate.*
$^*P < 0.05$ and $^{***}P < 0.001$ vs. the control (cited from [28]).*

expressed with α3β4 nAChRs, matsufushi extract and SJ-2 reversibly inhibited ACh (0.2 mM)-induced Na^+ currents (**Figure 6A, C**). Matsufushi extract (0.00003–0.001%) (**Figure 6B**) and SJ-2 (1–100 μM) (**Figure 6D**) significantly suppressed the Na^+ current in a concentration-dependent manner [27]. In addition, matsufushi and SJ-2 suppressed the ACh (0.3 mM)-induced ^{14}C-catecholamine synthesis from ^{14}C-tyrosine and tyrosine hydroxylase activity [27]. These results suggest that matsufushi extract inhibits ACh-induced catecholamine synthesis and secretion mainly due to SJ-2 via the suppression of Na^+ influx mediated through nAChR-ion channels [27].

4. Effects of the extract of sweet tea on catecholamine secretion and synthesis in adrenal medullary cells

Sweet tea is the processed leaves of *Hydrangea macrophylla* var. *thunbergii* Makino (hydrangeae dulcis folium), which is listed in the Japanese Pharmacopeia XV and used as a sweetening agent for diabetic patients. It also has antimicrobial and anti-allergic

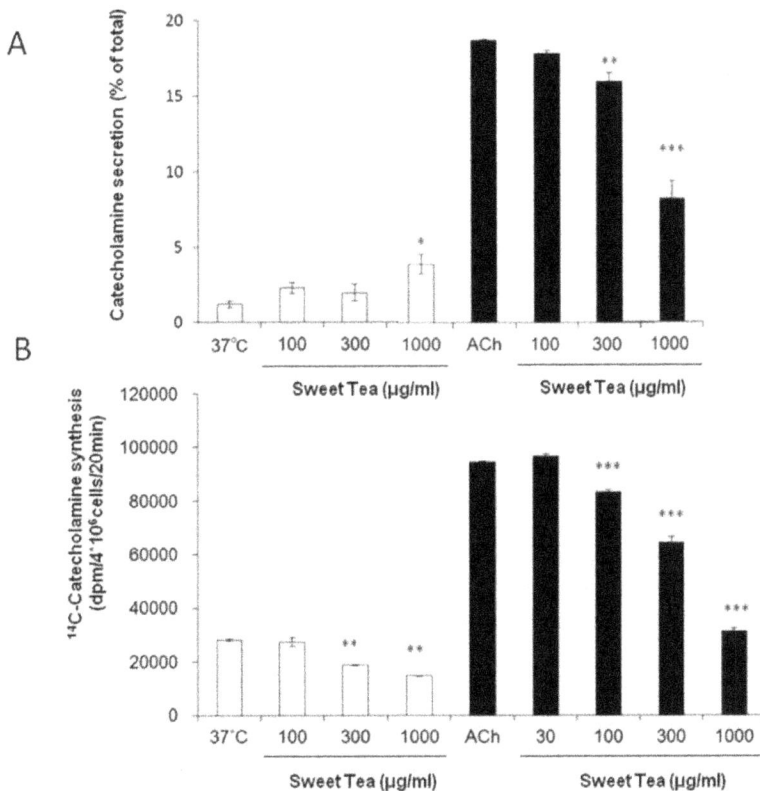

Figure 7.
*Effects of sweet tea on ^{14}C-catecholamine synthesis from [^{14}C]tyrosine (**A**) and tyrosine hydroxylase activity (**B**) in the cells. (**A**) Cells (4 × 10^6/dish) were incubated with L-[U-^{14}C] tyrosine (20 μM, 1 μCi) in the presence or absence of sweet tea (100–1000 μg/ml) and with or without 300-μM ACh at 37°C for 20 min. The ^{14}C-catecholamines formed were measured. (**B**) Cells (10^6/well) were incubated with L-[1-^{14}C] tyrosine (18 μM, 0.2 μCi) in the presence or absence of sweet tea (100–1000 μg/ml) and with or without 300 μM ACh at 37°C for 10 min, and tyrosine hydroxylase activity was measured. Data are means ± SEM from three separate experiments carried out in triplicate. $^*P < 0.05$, compared with 37°C (control), and $^{**}P < 0.01$ and $^{***}P < 0.001$ vs. ACh alone in (**A**), and $^{**}P < 0.01$ vs. 37°C (control) and $^{***}P < 0.001$ vs. ACh alone in (**B**).*

effects [30, 31]. Sweet tea is used as a healthy tea in Japan. There is, however, little evidence regarding sweet tea's effects on the sympathetic nervous system activity.

We investigated the effects of the extract of sweet tea on adrenal medullary cell function. A dry powder of sweet tea prepared from fermented leaves of hydrangeae dulcis folium was solubilized at 5.0 mg/ml and extracted at 90°C for 60 min. The extracted solution of sweet tea was used after centrifugation and filtration. The extract of sweet tea (1.0 mg/ml) slightly increased the basal secretion of catechol-amines (**Figure 7A**), whereas it suppressed the catecholamine secretion induced by ACh (0.3 mM) in a concentration-dependent manner (300–1000 μg/ml) (**Figure 7A**). In addition, the extract of sweet tea (300– or 100–1000 μg/ml) inhibited basal and ACh (0.3 mM)-induced ^{14}C-catecholamine synthesis from ^{14}C-tyrosine, respectively (**Figure 7B**). Sweet tea at concentrations of 3 mg/ml is usually used for drinking.

5. The insight of pharmacological potential of herbs in the catecholamine signaling induced by ACh in adrenal medulla

Adrenal medullary cells are derived from the embryonic neural crest and share many physiological and pharmacological properties with postganglionic sympathetic neurons [2]. The stimulation of AChRs in these cells increases the synthesis of catechol-amines and causes the secretion of catecholamines into the systemic circulation [2, 11, 14]. In adrenal medullary cells, the Na^+ influx induced by ACh via nAChR-ion channels is a prerequisite for Ca^{2+} influx via the activation of voltage-dependent Ca^{2+} channels and the subsequent catecholamine secretion and synthesis; in contrast, high K^+ directly gates voltage-dependent Ca^{2+} channels to increase $^{45}Ca^{2+}$ influx [2, 11] (**Figure 1**).

As we noted, ikarisoside A and matsufushi (or SJ-2) inhibited the catecholamine secretion induced by ACh, but not the secretion induced by 56 mM K^+ [10, 27]. In addition, ikarisoside A [10] and matsufushi [27] or SJ-2 [27] suppressed the Na^+ current induced by ACh in *Xenopus* oocytes expressing α3β4 nAChRs. These results suggest that the herbs and their components used as described herein inhibit the ACh-induced secretion and synthesis of catecholamines via a suppression of Na^+ influx mediated through nAChRs in adrenal medullary cells [10, 27].

It is well known that catecholamines have important roles in the regulation of normal function in the central and peripheral sympathetic nervous systems as a neurotransmitter but also in the adrenal medulla as an endocrine hormone [10]. Strong and prolonged stress causes massive amounts of catecholamine release, which can lead to cardiovascular diseases (such as hypertension, coronary heart disease, heart failure, and atherosclerosis), and such stress also suppresses the immune system to induce some cancers [2, 9, 10]. Indeed, chronic heart failure is associated with the activation of the sympathetic nervous system as manifested by an increased circulating level of noradrenaline and increased regional activity of the sympathetic nervous system [2, 32]. It was reported that the stress hormone adrenaline stimulates β2-adrenoceptors to activate the Gs-protein-dependent protein kinase A and the β-arrestin-1-mediated signaling pathway, which, in turn, suppresses p53 levels and triggers DNA damage [2, 33]. On the basis of these previous and present results, it appears that the herbs and their components such as ikarisoside A, matsufushi

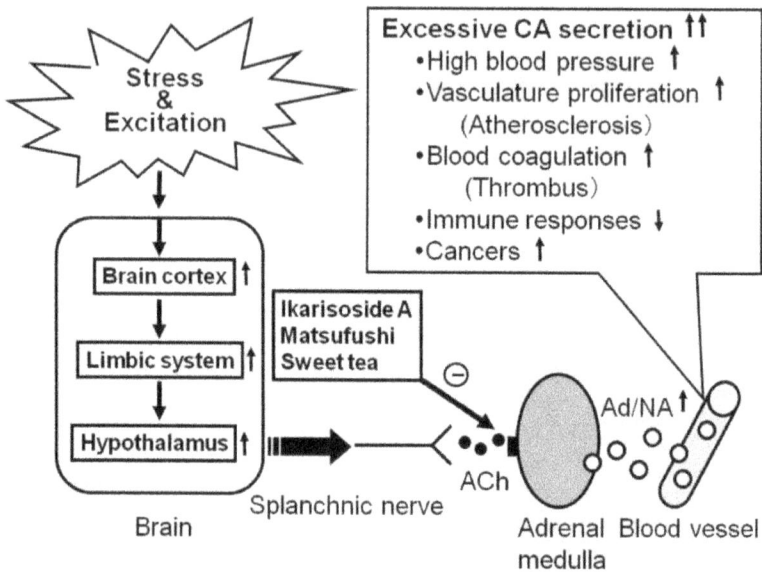

Figure 8.
Inhibitory mechanism of plant herbs (ikarisoside A, matsufushi, and sweet tea) on stress or excitation-induced excessive catecholamine secretion. Prolonged and strong stress or excitation stimulates the brain cortex, limbic system, and hypothalamus which evoke acetylcholine release from the splanchnic sympathetic nerves. Released acetylcholine induces a massive secretion of catecholamines from the adrenal medulla which may cause various deleterious symptoms or diseases such as high blood pressure (hypertension), vasculature proliferation (atherosclerosis), blood coagulation (thrombus), immune suppression, and cancers ([2] modified).

(or SJ-2), and sweet tea suppress the induction of a hyperactive catecholamine system induced by strong stress or emotional excitation (**Figure 8**).

6. Future perspective

Although the in vitro effects of the herbs and herb components described herein have been well clarified using cultured bovine adrenal medullary cells and *Xenopus* oocytes, the in vivo results are not yet clear. To confirm the pharmacological effects of these herbs on the catecholamine system, further in vivo studies of the effects of the administration of herbs to animals or humans are needed [2, 27]. We observed a disturbance of the autonomic nervous balance in women with climacteric symptoms measured by a power spectral analysis of heart rate variability [34]. Using this assay method, we will examine the effect of herbs on the autonomic nervous activity under some stress conditions.

7. Concluding remarks

We have reviewed the evidence that herbs and their components such as ikarisoside A, matsufushi (or SJ-2), and sweet tea inhibit the catecholamine synthesis and secretion induced by ACh in cultured bovine adrenal medullary cells and summarized them in **Table 1**. These findings may provide new insights into the pharmacological potentials of herbs on the hyperactive catecholamine system induced by stress.

Herb	Epimedium	Pine nodule	Sweet tea
Supplement	+	+	+
Compound	Ikarisoside A	SJ-2	ND
ACh-induced Na$^+$ current	↓	↓	ND
ACh-induced Ca^{2+} influx	↓	↓	ND
Catecholamine secretion			
Basal	→	→	↑
ACh-induced	↓	↓	↓
Catecholamine synthesis			
Basal	→	→	↓
ACh-induced	↓	↓	↓

Supplement +, available in Japan; ND, not determined.

Table 1.
Summary of the effects of herbs and their components on catecholamine secretion and synthesis.

Conflict of interest

The authors have no conflict of interest to declare.

Funding

This work was supported, in part, by Grant-in-Aid (26350170) for Scientific Research (C) from the Japan Society for the Promotion of Science and Grant-in-Aid

(160701 and 170701) for Health Labor Sciences Research Grant and by Tokujun Co. (Kobe, Japan) and Nozaki Kampo Pharmacy (Gifu, Japan).

Abbreviations

ACh	acetylcholine
nAChR	nicotinic acetylcholine receptor

Author details

Nobuyuki Yanagihara[1,2*], Xiaoja Li[3], Yumiko Toyohira[2], Noriaki Satoh[4], Hui Shao[5], Yasuhiro Nozaki[6], Shin Ishikane[2], Fumi Takahashi[2], Ryo Okada[7], Hideyuki Kobayashi[7], Masato Tsutsui[8] and Taizo Kita[9]

1 Laboratory of Pharmacology, Faculty of Food and Nutrition, Kyushu Nutrition Welfare University, Kitakyushu, Japan

2 Department of Pharmacology, University of Occupational and Environmental Health, School of Medicine, Kitakyushu, Japan

3 Institute for Environmental and Gender-Specific Medicine, Graduate School of Medicine, Juntendo University, Urayasu, Japan

4 Shared-Use Research Center, Facility for Education and Research Support, University of Occupational and Environmental Health, Kitakyushu, Japan

5 Tokujun Pharmaceutical Research Institute, Kobe, Japan

6 Nozaki Kanpo Pharmacy, Gifu, Japan

7 Department of Chemistry, University of Occupational and Environmental Health, School of Medicine, Kitakyushu, Japan

8 Department of Pharmacology, Graduate School of Medicine, University of the Ryukyus, Okinawa, Japan

9 Offices under the President, Setsunan University, Neyagawa, Japan

*Address all correspondence to: yanagin@knwu.ac.jp

IntechOpen

© 2018 The Author(s). Licensee IntechOpen. This chapter is distributed under the terms of the Creative Commons Attribution License (http://creativecommons.org/licenses/by/3.0), which permits unrestricted use, distribution, and reproduction in any medium, provided the original work is properly cited. (cc) BY

References

[1] Lu MF, Xiao ZT, Zhang HY. Where do health benefits of flavonoids come from? Insights from flavonoid targets and their evolutionary history. Biochemical and Biophysical Research Communications. 2013;**434**(4):701-704

[2] Yanagihara N, Zhang H, Toyohira Y, Takahashi K, Ueno S, Tsutsui M, et al. New insights into the pharmacological potential of plant flavonoids in the catecholamine system. Journal of Pharmacological Sciences. 2014;**124**:123-128

[3] Nijveldt RJ, van Nood E, van Hoorn DE, Boelens PG, van Norren K, van Leeuwen PA. Flavonoids: A review of probable mechanisms of action and potential applications. The American Journal of Clinical Nutrition. 2001;**74**(4):418-425

[4] Ren ZL, Zuo PP. Neural regeneration: Role of traditional Chinese medicine in neurological diseases treatment. Journal of Pharmacological Sciences. 2012;**120**(3):139-145

[5] Falcone Ferreyra ML, Rius SP, Casati P. Flavonoids: Biosynthesis, biological functions, and biotechnological applications. Frontiers in Plant Science. 2012;**3**:222

[6] Gehm BD, McAndrews JM, Chien P-Y, Jameson JL. Resveratrol, a polyphenolic compound found in grapes and wine, is an agonist for the estrogen receptor. Proceedings of the National Academy of Sciences of the United States of America. 1997;**94**:14138-14143

[7] Wu JM, Wang ZR, Hsieh TC, Bruder JL, Zou JG, Huang YZ. Mechanism of cardioprotection by resveratrol, a phenolic antioxidant present in red wine (Review). International Journal of Molecular Medicine. 2001;**8**:3-17

[8] Renaud S, de Lorgeril M. Wine, alcohol, platelets, and the French Paradox for coronary heart disease. Lancet. 1992;**339**:1523-1526

[9] Westfall TC, Westfall DP. Neurotransmission: The autonomic and somatic motor nervous systems. In: Brunton LL, Chabner B, Knollman B, editors. Goodman & Gilman's the Pharmacological Basis of Therapeutics. 12th ed. New York: McGraw-Hill; 2011. pp. 171-218

[10] Li X, Toyohira Y, Horisita T, Satoh N, Takahashi K, Zhang H, et al. Ikarisoside A inhibits acetylcholine-induced catecholamine secretion and synthesis by suppressing nicotinic acetylcholine receptor-ion channels in cultured bovine adrenal medullary cells. Naunyn-Schmiedeberg's Archives of Pharmacology. 2015;**388**:1259-1269

[11] Wada A, Takara H, Izumi F, Kobayashi H, Yanagihara N. Influx of ^{22}Na through acetylcholine receptor-associated Na channels: relationship between ^{22}Na influx, ^{45}Ca influx and secretion of catecholamines in cultured bovine adrenal medulla cells. Neuroscience. 1985;**15**(1):283-292

[12] Yanagihara N, Tank AW, Weiner N. Relationship between activation and phosphorylation of tyrosine hydroxylase by 56 mm K$^+$ in PC12 cells in culture. Molecular Pharmacology. 1984;**26**:141-147

[13] Yanagihara N, Tank AW, Langan TA, Weiner N. Enhanced phosphorylation of tyrosine hydroxylase at more than one site is induced by 56 mM K$^+$ in rat pheochromocytoma PC12 cells in culture. Journal of Neurochemistry. 1986;**46**:562-568

[14] Yanagihara N, Wada A, Izumi F. Effects of α_2-adrenergic agonists on carbachol-stimulated catecholamine

synthesis in cultured bovine adrenal medullary cells. Biochemical Pharmacology. 1987;**36**:3823-3828

[15] Tachikawa E, Tank AW, Yanagihara N, Mosimann W, Weiner N. Phosphorylation of tyrosine hydroxylase on at least three sites in rat pheochromocytoma PC12 cells treated with 56 mM K$^+$: determination of the sites on tyrosine hydroxylase phosphorylated by cyclic AMP-dependent and calcium/calmodulin-dependent protein kinases. Molecular Pharmacology. 1986;**30**:476-485

[16] Yoshimura R, Yanagihara N, Hara K, Nakamura J, Toyohira Y, Ueno S, et al. Dual phases of functional changes in norepinephrine transporter in cultured bovine adrenal medullary cells by long-term treatment with clozapine. Journal of Neurochemistry. 2001;**77**:1018-1026

[17] Kajiwara K, Yanagita T, Nakashima Y, Wada A, Izumi F, Yanagihara N. Differential effects of short and prolonged exposure to carvedilol on voltage-dependent Na$^+$ channels in cultured bovine adrenal medullary cells. The Journal of Pharmacology and Experimental Therapeutics. 2002;**302**:212-218

[18] Obara G, Toyohira Y, Inagaki H, Takahashi K, Horishita T, Kawasaki T, et al. Pentazocine inhibits norepinephrine transporter function by reducing its surface expression in bovine adrenal medullary cells. Journal of Pharmacological Sciences. 2013;**121**(2):138-147

[19] Liu M, Yanagihara N, Toyohira Y, Tsutsui M, Ueno S, Shinohara Y. Dual effects of daidzein, a soy isoflavone, on catecholamine synthesis and secretion in cultured bovine adrenal medullary cells. *Endocrinologie*. 2007;**148**:5348-5354

[20] Toyohira Y, Ueno S, Tsutsui M, Itho H, Sakai N, Saito N, et al. Stimulatory effects of the soy phytoestrogen genistein on noradrenaline transporter and serotonin transporter activity. Molecular Nutrition & Food Research. 2010;**54**:516-524

[21] Zhang H, Toyohira Y, Ueno S, Shinohara Y, Itoh H, Furuno Y, et al. Dual effects of nobiletin, a citrus polymethoxy flavone, on catecholamine secretion in cultured bovine adrenal medullary cells. Journal of Neurochemistry. 2010;**114**:1030-1038

[22] Shinohara Y, Toyohira Y, Ueno S, Liu M, Tsutsui M, Yanagihara N. Effects of resveratrol, a grape polyphenol, on catecholamine secretion and synthesis in cultured bovine adrenal medullary cells. Biochemical Pharmacology. 2007;**74**:1608-1618

[23] Dou J, Liu Z, Liu S. Structure identification of a prenylflavonol glycoside from Epimedium koreanum by electrospray ionization tandem mass spectrometry. Analytical Sciences. 2006;**22**:449-452

[24] Choi HJ, Eun JS, Park YR, Kim DK, Li R, Moon WS, et al. Ikarisoside A inhibits inducible nitric oxide synthase in lipopolysaccharide-stimulated RAW 264.7 cells via p38 kinase and nuclear factor-kB signaling pathways. European Journal of Pharmacology. 2008;**601**:171-178

[25] Choi HJ, Park YR, Nepal M, Choi BY, Cho NP, Choi SH, et al. Inhibition of osteoclastogenic differentiation by Ikarisoside A in RAW 264.7 cells via JNK and NF-kB signaling pathways. European Journal of Pharmacology. 2010;**636**:28-35

[26] Li C, Li Q, Mei Q, Lu T. Pharmacological effects and pharmacokinetic properties of icariin, the major bioactive component in Herba Epimedii. Life Sciences. 2015;**126**:57-68

[27] Li X, Horisita T, Toyohira Y, Shao H, Bai J, Bo H, et al. Inhibitory effects of pine nodule extract and its component, SJ-2, on acetylcholine-induced catecholamine secretion and synthesis in bovine adrenal medullary cells. Journal of Pharmacological Sciences. 2017;**133**:268-275

[28] Bermudez J, Burgess MF, Cassidy F, Clarke GD. Activity of the oxidation of products of oleum terebinthinae "Landes" on guinea pig airway smooth muscle in vivo and in vitro. Arzneimittel-Forschung. 1987;**37**:1258-1262

[29] Chen W, Liu Y, Li M, Mao J, Zhang L, Huang R. Anti-tumor effect of α-pinene on human hepatoma cell lines through inducing G2/M cell cycle arrest. Journal of Pharmacological Sciences. 2015;**127**:332-338

[30] Yoshikawa M, Harada E, Naitoh Y, Inoue K, Matsuda H, Shimoda H, et al. Development of bioactive functions in hydrangeae dulcis folium. III. On the antiallergic and antimicrobial principles of hydrangeae dulcis folium. (1). Thunberginols A, B, and F. Chemical & Pharmaceutical Bulletin (Tokyo). 1994;**42**:2225-2230

[31] Wang Q, Matsuda H, Matsuhira K, Nakamura S, Yuan D, Yoshikawa M. Inhibitory effects of thunberginols A, B, and F on degranulations and releases of TNF-alpha and IL-4 in RBL-2H3 cells. Chemical & Pharmaceutical Bulletin (Tokyo). 2007;**30**:388-392

[32] Freedman NJ, Lefkowitz RJ. Anti-β_1-adrenergic receptor antibodies and heart failure: causation, not just correlation. The Journal of Clinical Investigation. 2004;**113**:1379-1382

[33] Hara MR, Kovacs JJ, Whalen EJ, Rajagopal S, Strachan RT, Grant W, et al. A stress response pathway regulates DNA damage through β_2-adrenoreceptors and β-arrestin-1. Nature. 2011;**477**(7364):349-353

[34] Yanagihara N, Seki M, Nakano M, Hachisuga T, Goto Y. An inverse correlation between cardiac vagal activity and the simplified menopause index in Japanese menopausal climacteric women. Menopause. 2014;**21**:669-672

Chapter 5

Thrombotic Tendencies in Excess Catecholamine States

Vivek K. Nambiar and Drisya Rajan Chalappurath

Abstract

Catecholamines are neurotransmitters distributed throughout the body including adrenal glands, chromaffin tissues and other tissues innervated by post ganglionic adrenergic neurons. The rate of release of medullary hormones is responsible for the control of serum catecholamines. Thrombogenicity of catecholamines are due various mechanisms including hypercoagulable states, endothelial damage, blood stasis and platelet aggregation. Oxidative stress generated by catecholamine excess causes coronary spasm, ultrastructural cell damage and arrhythmias. Elevated plasminogen activator inhibitor-1 during catecholamine excess causes hypercoagulability by hypofibrinosis. During stress, Catecholamines released in procoagulant environment causes vasoconstriction in adrenal veins resulting in venous thrombosis. Catecholamines generate moderately elevated levels of platelet count which enhances the risk of thrombosis. Hypercoagulability results in formation of coronary thrombus, rupture of atherosclerotic plaque and plaque progression due to gradual fibrinogen accumulation in the vessel walls. High levels of circulating catecholamines produce elevated levels thrombomodulin, the biomarkers of endothelial cell damage. In patients with hypertension in catecholamine excess, resistance to blood flow and damage to the integrity of blood vessels lead to atherosclerosis. A case report has been discussed which suggests an association of thrombotic tendency and catecholamine excess.

Keywords: catecholamines, thrombotic tendencies, atherosclerosis, hypercoagulation, platelet aggregation, endothelial damage, blood stasis

1. Introduction

Catecholamines are the class of neurotransmitters and hormones produced by the adrenergic nervous system, with a core structure of catechol and an amine group, regulating physiological processes [1]. Catechol refers to *ortho-dihydroxybenzene* and epinephrine and norepinephrine are the two major ethanolamine derivatives [2] occurring in the blood [3]. About 80% of epinephrine and 20% of norepinephrine are produced and released by the human adrenal medulla with a small amount of dopamine along with it [2].

1.1 Catecholamine biosynthesis

Catecholamines are synthesised and secreted from the chromaffin cells in adrenal medulla and sympathetic paraganglia [4]. Chromaffin granules produce catecholamines and fairly high concentration of adenosine triphosphate (ATP) and adenosine diphosphate (ADP) for active transport mechanism [2].

IntechOpen

Syntheses of catecholamines occur at two levels [5]:

1. Sympathetic nervous fibre extremities for norepinephrine.

2. Chromaffin cells of adrenal medulla for both epinephrine and norepinephrine.

Tyrosine hydroxylase is the rate limiting enzyme of catecholamine synthesis. Tyrosine from dietary proteins is transported to the brain and tyrosine hydroxylase (in the dopaminergic and noradrenergic neurons of CNS and in the non-neuronal cells of gastrointestinal tract and kidneys) converts it to 3,4-dihydroxyphenylala-nine (DOPA). In the presence of aromatic L-amino acid decarboxylase, DOPA is converted to dopamine (DA) which is transported to vesicular storage granules. It may be released in the dopaminergic neurons or converted to norepinephrine in the noradrenergic neurons by dopamine beta-hydroxylase [6]. Norepinephrine is converted to epinephrine by phenyl ethanolamine-N-methyltransferase (PNMT) [4].

Medullary hormones synthesised and stored in the chromaffin granules are a pool of ready to release hormones upon stimulation [7].

1.2 Catecholamine functions and receptors

Norepinephrine and epinephrine together contribute to an increase in cardiac output, heart-rate, respiration, blood pressure, blood flow to muscles, alertness and decrease in splanchnic and renal blood flow [2]. Norepinephrine alone causes a decrease in heart-rate indirectly as a result of reflex bradycardia because of vaso-constriction effects [2].

Functions of catecholamines are mediated and regulated by alpha, beta adreno-receptors and dopamine receptors. Each receptor located at distinct locations serves different functions and actions.

Alpha-1 receptors mediate adrenergic vasoconstriction [8]. Alpha-2 receptor stimulation causes inhibition of norepinephrine secretion [6]. Three subtypes of α_2 receptors are α_{2A}, α_{2B}, and α_{2C}. Alpha-2A in the peripheral postsynaptic region contributes to vasoconstriction in different vascular beds [8]. Beta-1 receptor stimulation causes positive inotropic and chronotropic action [6]. Beta-2 receptors stimulate vasodilation [9]. Beta 3 causes lipolysis in fatty cells and increase renin secretion [9].

Two types of dopamine receptors are D1 and D2.Stimulation of D1 receptors in coronary, renal, mesenteric and cerebrovascular beds causes vasodilation, diuresis and natriuresis. D2 receptor stimulation in presynaptic nerve endings causes inhibition of norepinephrine release [6].

1.3 Catecholamine metabolism

Neuronal catecholamines get metabolised intraneuronally after leakage from its stores [1]. Catecholamine metabolism mainly occurs in the liver [2]. There are two major catecholamine metabolites (i) metanephrines (constitutes 15% of urinary catecholamine) and (ii) vanillylmandelic acid, VMA (major end-point of norepinephrine and epinephrine metabolism [1] and constitutes 85% of excreted catecholamine) [2].

1.4 Catecholamine inactivation

Two major enzymes involved in the inactivation of catecholamines are catechol-o-methyl transferase (COMT) and monoamine oxidase (MAO).COMT adds methyl group to hydroxyl at 3-position of catechol ring and MAO catalyses oxidative deamination reaction [2].

Norepinephrine is inactivated by two processes (i) reuptake into the nerve terminals by the active carrier mechanism associated with Na^+-K^+-ATPase of which some part is stored to granular vesicles and the rest is metabolised and (ii) extra-neuronal accumulation to vascular smooth muscles [10].

1.5 Catecholamine excess

The three distinct peripheral catecholamine systems are [11].

1. Sympathetic nervous system (SNS)

2. Adrenomedullary hormone system (AHS)

3. Dopamine autocrine/paracrine system (DOPA)

Sympathetic nervous system: the measure of norepinephrine release in the specific regions allows the clinical assessment of organ-specific sympathetic nervous tone and penetrating analysis of SNS in the pathophysiology of a disease state [12].

Adrenomedullary hormone system: the catecholamines stored in the chromaffin cells get released by innervations of preganglionic sympathetic fibres of splanchnic nerves and get dispersed after its entry to medulla [2].

Dopamine derived from plasma DOPA acts as an autocrine/paracrine substance. Human urine contains higher concentration of dopamine and its metabolites rather than norepinephrine and its metabolites as dopamine is generated in the non-noradrenergic and non-adrenergic cells [13].

Catecholamines are distributed throughout the body including adrenal glands, chromaffin tissues and other tissues innervated by post ganglionic adrenergic neurons [3]. The rate of release of medullary hormones is responsible for the control of serum catecholamines [2].

The cellular uptake and metabolism of catecholamines in the extraneuronal tissues and the exogenous administration of catecholamines together contribute to 25% of total metabolism of catecholamines produced in the SNS and adrenergic chromaffin cells [1].

During stressful conditions, the level of enzymes catalysing biosynthesis of catecholamines increase and enzymes degrading the catecholamines decrease [14]. Stress-induced changes in the adrenergic receptors occur due to the combination of neuronal and extraneuronal catecholamine uptake system, level of cAMP, density of adrenoceptor subtypes and coupling of agonist receptor complex with different G-proteins [14].

During chronic stress, increased levels of catecholamines produce aminolutins and oxyradicals. Oxidative stress thus generated causes coronary spasm, ultrastructural cell damage and arrhythmias [14]. They also cause Ca^{2+} overload and cardiac dysfunction by acting on beta-1-adrenoceptor signal transduction pathway [14].

1.6 Catecholamine excess in pheochromocytoma

Catecholamine excess is seen in certain types of tumour such as pheochromocytomas that are functional tumours of the chromaffin cells [15]. Norepinephrine secreting tumours are known to cause hypertension (in 80–90% of these patients [4]) and hypertensive crisis and their abrupt release may cause arrhythmias [6]. Of this nearly 40% of the patients suffer from sustained hypertension (norepinephrine secreting tumours), 45% from paroxysmal hypertension (epinephrine secreting tumours) and 5–15% from normotension (dopamine secreting tumours) [4].

Other vasoactive substances like neuropeptide Y, adrenomedullin and atrial natriuretic peptide contribute to hypertension in these patients [6]. Neuropeptide Y increase coronary and peripheral vascular resistance and potentiate norepinephrine-induced vasoconstriction [7].

Pheochromocytoma produces enormous amounts of catecholamines due to mutation of succinate dehydrogenase by oxidative phosphorylation deficit [6].Two major mechanisms in pheochromocytoma that leads to catecholamine excess are translocation of dopamine into storage granules and the presence of dopamine beta hydroxylase enzyme [1].

In extra-adrenal tumours, norepinephrine levels are high, in adrenal tumours both norepinephrine and epinephrine are in excess and in multiple endocrine neoplasia type 2 and neurofibromatosis type 1, epinephrine levels are high [6].

In non-functional/silent pheochromocytoma, metanephrine levels are elevated instead of catecholamines [6].

Complication of pheochromocytoma in hypertensive crisis are sustained hypertension by continuous elevated levels of catecholamine causing vasoconstriction and orthostatic hypertension due to reduced blood volume that resulting in vasoconstriction, postural tachycardia and postural hypotension [4].

Neurological complications are hypertensive encephalopathy, haemorrhage (due to paroxysmal hypertension) and acute ischemic stroke (due to postural hypertension) [4].

In 78% of pheochromocytoma patients, thrombus exists at the time of their tumour discovery and 75% of the secondary thrombi are located in inferior vena cava or heart or both [16]. Venous thromboembolism and acute arterial thrombi are well described in such patients [17] but evidence of stroke, aortic thrombi and myocardial infarction are fewer [18].

Several mechanisms explain thrombotic tendencies in pheochromocytomas by elevated catecholamines:

- Catecholamines generate moderately elevated levels of platelet count which enhance the risk of thrombosis [19].

- Platelet aggregation is increased in pheochromocytoma [18] and produce thrombi in low-flow areas causing coronary events [19].

- Contributing factors to thrombus formation are erythropoietin, pro-coagulation and serotonin [6].

- Catecholamine excess in other tumours like paragangliomas may cause ADP-mediated platelet aggregation leading to thrombotic events [20].

- During stress, catecholamine release in procoagulant environment causes vasoconstriction in adrenal veins resulting in venous thrombosis [21].

- Loss of antithrombin III in glomerular diseases associated with hypertension may increase thrombotic risk [22].

- Pheochromocytoma causes thrombosis of caudal vena cava and aortic thromboembolism through Virchow's triad list [20, 22]:

(i) Endothelial damage

(ii) Blood stasis

(iii) Hypercoagulability state

Mortality of pheochromocytoma patients occur due to either acute intramyocardial necrosis or diffuse patchy myocardial fibrosis [23].

2. Mechanisms associated with thrombus formation in catecholamine excess

Thrombus formation and dissolution are physiological processes with dynamic balance between procoagulation and anticoagulation mechanism [24]. Catecholamine excess contributes to long-term development of atherosclerosis and cardiovascular risk [25] due to their effect on carbohydrate and lipid metabolism [23].

3. Cascade of thrombus formation

Thrombotic process occurs by the activation of coagulation cascade in different phases [26].

1. Initiation phase—the extrinsic pathway of coagulation in which low amounts of active pro-coagulant factors are produced.

2. Amplification phase—level of coagulation factors increase.

3. Propagation phase—active coagulation factors are generated like thrombin which binds to phospholipid at the surface of activated platelets.

4. Stabilization phase—thrombin provides strength and stability to growing clot and thrombin activatable fibrinolysis inhibitor.

Injury to the vessel walls due to resistance, in catecholamine excess states, causes exposure of glycoprotein tissue factor (TF) to the blood. After exposure, TF bind to Factor VII/VIIa and forms tertiary complex in the presence of calcium to activate factor X to Xa, factor IX to IXa and factor VIIa. At the site of injury, platelet activation, conversion of fibrinogen to fibrin and thrombus formation occurs. Platelets are able to regulate their gene and protein expression for binding to sub endothelium [26].

Diseases affecting Virchow's triad can induce clot formation [27].

4. Hypercoagulability

Hypercoagulability is the tendency to produce thrombosis by inherited or acquired molecular defects. Thrombus is formed based on the number of predisposing factors and environmental stress [13].

Cancer is the second major cause of hypercoagulation with clinical thrombosis in 15% and thrombosis on autopsy in 50% patients [28].

Catecholamines increase plasminogen activator inhibitor-1 (PAI-1) mRNA by expression of PAI-1 genes in the cardiovascular system by neurological and neuro-endocrine mechanisms via beta-adrenoreceptors [29]. PAI-1, a member of serine-protease inhibitor, inhibits both tissue type and urinary-type plasminogen activator. Elevated PAI-1 during catecholamine excess causes hypercoagulability by hypofi-brinosis. High levels of PAI-1 act on adipokines in the atherogenic process and cause atherosclerotic lesions and atheromas [30]. Epinephrine regulates Beta-mediated tissue-type plasminogen activator to produce an increase in fibrinolytic capacity [25].

Antithrombin III (AT-III) inhibits the protein-splitting reaction, characteristic of haemostasis, by interfering with the activity of four of the serine proteases and antagonising thrombin [31]. Hypertension associated glomerular diseases in catecholamine excess may cause loss of AT-III by protein loss in the urine. Hypoalbuminemia and hypercholesterolemia in Proteinuria causes platelet hyper-aggregability and aggravate hypercoagulability. Increased levels of fibrinogen and thromboxane in protein-losing nephropathy contribute to thrombosis [27].

Hypercoagulability result in formation of coronary thrombus, rupture of ath-erosclerotic plaque and plaque progression due to gradual fibrinogen accumulation in the vessel walls [24].

In patients with borderline hypertension, coagulation activation occurs before clinical manifestations of vascular damage appear [32].

5. Platelet aggregation

In thrombus formation, a high proportion of platelets translocates from their initial point of attachment to the injured vessel wall and forms a firm adhesion contact [31]. Catecholamine infusion induces platelet aggregation in ex-vivo and animal models [16]. They activate platelets by interacting with platelet α2-adrenoreceptor in in-vitro studies. Stimulation of α1-adrenoreceptor inhibits platelet aggregation by inactivating platelet response to epinephrine [25]. In-vivo adrenergic infusion causes platelet activation and an increase in platelet size, aggregation and releasing factors [24]. Elevated factor V: C, factor VIII: C, v Willebrand Factor: Ag, tissue-plasminogen activator (t-PA): Ag, contribute to risk of atherothrombotic events [25]. Redistribution of cardiac blood flow in catechol-amine infusion causes regional slowing of blood flow and enhanced tendency for intravascular platelet aggregation [23].

The anticoagulative effect of epinephrine is explained by a 50% decrease in the ratio of maximal coagulation activation and maximal fibrinolytic activa-tion by decreased tumour necrosis factor (TNF) and interleukin (IL) 10 [33]. Epinephrine induce fibrinogen receptor exposure and fibrinogen binding to potentiate platelet aggregation. Epinephrine infusion causes short-term recruit-ment of platelets and functionally active Factor VIII from the spleen for thrombus formation. They discharge high molecular von Willebrand Factor (vWF) which increase the activity of platelet adhesion from its storage compartments. Elevated epinephrine levels increase platelet deposition on the atherosclerotic vessels with high local shear rate [25].

Norepinephrine activates platelet aggregation in-vivo by stimulating α2-adrenoreceptor [24].

It causes platelet aggregation in two phases [16]:

• Initial reversible aggregation.

• Simulated release of adenosine diphosphate.

Norepinephrine initiates platelet thrombosis by directly damaging the endothelial walls of vessels and breaking its integrity [24]. In acute mental stress, 60% of variation in thrombin formation depends on amount of norepinephrine secreted and sensitivity of β2-adrenergic receptor [19].

6. Clotting time

Adrenergic activation by epinephrine injection increases factor VIII: C and cause a decrease in clotting time. In-vivo adrenergic infusion stimulate β-2 adrenergic vascular receptors to release clotting factors like FVIII, v WF, and t-PA from endothelium to the circulation [24] resulting in thrombotic risk in both coronary artery disease and hypertension [25].

7. Endothelial damage

Endothelium maintains balance between prothrombotic and atherothrombotic tendencies [27]. Endothelial cells provide a non-thrombogenic surface that inhibits platelets and blood cells from adhering and activating coagulation cascade [34]. Antithrombotics like thrombomodulin, heparin sulfate, tissue factor pathway inhibitor and protein S are involved in reducing the activation of AT III and protein c to elevate antithrombotic tendencies. Synthesis and induction of prothrombotic mediators such as tissue factor and antifibrinolytic factors like PAI-1 take part in prothrombotic tendencies [27].

Disproportion in the tendencies causes endothelial damage where subendothelial proteins are exposed and favour platelet adhesion [27]. According to Gando et al. [35], endothelial damage can occur due to both exogenous and endogenous release of catecholamines. High levels of circulating catecholamines produce elevated levels thrombomodulin, the biomarkers of endothelial cell damage [36]. Due to loss of endothelial cell protection and expression of pro-coagulant and prothrombotic molecules, platelets adhere to the subendothelial surface and release ADP and thromboxane A2 causing imbalance in haemostasis and thrombosis [37].

8. Blood stasis

Blood stasis plays an important role in the formation of thrombus. Thrombus forms in regions of blood stasis like narrow artery due to atheromatous plaque, mechanical vasoconstriction, prolonged immobilisation and varicose vein. From the injured tissue, tissue thromboplastin produced causes initial thrombus formation followed by platelet activation by thrombin. Thrombin transforms fibrinogen to insoluble fibrin and release to stagnant blood [36].

In patients with hypertension in catecholamine excess, resistance to blood flow and damage to the integrity of blood vessels lead to atherosclerosis [27, 32]. Three mechanisms explain the overall increased vascular resistance [37]:

(i) Rarefaction of arterioles and capillaries.

(ii) Reduced internal diameter of arterioles.

(iii) Increase in arterial and arteriolar wall mass.

S. No.	Mechanism of thrombosis	Factors involved in thrombosis
1.	Hypercoagulability	1. Tissue plasminogen activator inhibitor-1 (t-PAI-1) 2. Antithrombin-III (AT-III) 3. Fibrinogen 4. Thromboxane
2.	Platelet aggregation	1. Factor V: C 2. Factor VIII: C 3. v Willebrand factor (v WF) 4. t-PAI-1 5. Tumour necrosis factor (TNF) 6. Interleukin 10 (IL-10)
3.	Clotting time	1. Factor VIII:C 2. (v WF) 3. t-PAI-1
4.	Endothelial damage	1. t-PAI-1 2. Thrombomodulin 3. Thromboxane A2
5.	Blood stasis	1. Thromboplastin 2. Thrombin

Table 1.
Summary of factors associated with thrombosis.

The significant role of sympathetic nervous system in elevated haemostatic activity in atherosclerosis and thrombus formation explains the role of catecholamines in cardiovascular diseases and associated arterial thrombus formation [25]. The factors associated with thrombosis in different mechanisms are summarised in **Table 1**.

9. Management of thrombosis

Hypertension associated with catecholamine excess plays an important role in the thrombus formation by mechanisms explained above. So treatment for hypertension is the primary objective in treatment and prevention of thrombotic tendencies. The most preferred antihypertensive is phenoxybenzamine which is an alpha and beta receptor antagonist given at 10 mg once a day with gradual dose titration to 30 mg three times a day. Appropriate anti-coagulation with heparin is vital for patients with risk of thrombosis to prevent devastating outcomes [19].

Removal of tumours producing excess catecholamines play a crucial role in alleviating symptoms associated with hypertension and thus thrombus formation. Due exaggerated fall in blood pressure after surgical removal of these tumours, adequate vascular volume replacement with oral fluids and salt is recommended [38].

Here in a case report has been discussed which suggests an association of thrombotic tendency and catecholamine excess.

10. Case report

A Case report on cerebral venous thrombosis due to pheochromocytoma in a patient with Von Hippel Lindau (VHL) mutation [39] explains an unusual connection between thrombosis and pheochromocytoma in a 15 year old boy with pheochromocytoma and associated hypertension. The patient was primarily presented with cerebral venous thrombosis and seizures. Initial examination revealed left frontoparietal hematoma and superior sagittal and transverse sinus thrombus for which he was treated with heparin and antiepileptics. Follow-up showed elevated blood pressure and high urine catecholamine levels. The diagnosis of abdominal mass after evaluation for consistent elevated blood pressure turned out to be pheochromocytoma. He underwent para-aortic dissection and right adrenalectomy.

VHL disease is an autosomal, dominant inherited tumour syndrome which occurs as a result of a germline mutation in the VHL gene. Even though its association with pheochromocytoma is under-studied, VHL proteins are found to cause tumorigenesis in pheochromocytoma by induction of either gain of function, dominant negative effect or gene dosage effect in chromaffin cells [40].

Some mechanisms are established to explain the association of Catecholamine excess in pheochromocytoma and thrombus formation:

1. Tumours produce different chemicals with prothrombotic nature that cause hypercoagulability as a paraneoplastic feature [41]. The release of procoagulants, fibrinolytics and proteolytic factors induce thrombosis. Neoplastic vascular invasion damages the thromboresistant properties of vessel wall and tumour cell attachment to the endothelial surface leading to endothelial retraction and exposure of basement membrane. The damaged endothelial cells and matrix cause platelet adhesion and aggregation by release of procoagulatory and antagonistic substances [42].

2. Adrenal tumours release excess catecholamines and cause thrombophilia and clot formation [16].

3. In the case of VHL mutation, certain changes are produced in the Hypoxia inducible factor (HIF) resulting in polycythaemia and increased venous thrombosis [43]. HIF regulates both oxygen hemostasis and erythropoietin receptor expression [44, 45].

To associate hereditary disorders with thrombosis in excess catecholamine state is restricted because of unavailability of literatures explaining the same. Excess catecholamines themselves produce thrombosis even though an inherent mutation of VHL was found in the above patient as a cause of thrombosis. Hypertension associated with high catecholamine levels make a patient more prone to thrombosis than others with normal blood pressure. In patients with tumours such as pheochromocytoma and paraganglioma, there is high catecholamine levels which increase the risk of thrombotic tendencies compared to other patients with catecholamine excess alone.

11. Conclusion

Though there have been evidences of thrombus formation after infusion of catecholamines in animals and humans, available evidence of the exact mechanism of thrombotic tendencies is scanty. Catecholamine excess states are a diagnostic challenge due to heterogenous clinical presentation like fluctuating hypertension in young which may not attract enough clinical and laboratory attention. Thrombogenicity of catecholamines are due various mechanisms including hypercoagulable states, endothelial damage, blood stasis and platelet aggregation. Surgical removal of tumours associated with catecholamine excess provide a clinical approach in treating abnormalities of thrombus formation.

Acknowledgements

We express our gratitude towards Amrutha Ajai and Sharon Ann Georgy for their editorial support.

Conflict of interest

There are no conflicts of interest.

Abbreviations

ADP	adenosine diphosphate
ATP	adenosine triphosphate
DOPA	3,4-dihydroxyphenylalanine
DA	dopamine
PNMT	phenyl ethanolamine-N-methyl transferase
COMT	catechol-O-methyl transferase
MAO	monoamine oxidase
SNS	sympathetic nervous system
ANS	autonomic nervous system
DOPA	dopamine autocrine/paracrine system
PAI-1	plasminogen activator inhibitor-1
AT-III	antithrombin III
t-PA	tissue plasminogen activator
TNF	tumour necrosis factor
IL	interleukin
v WF	von Willebrand factor
VHL	Von Hippel Lindau
HIF	hypoxia inducible factor

Author details

Vivek K. Nambiar[1] and Drisya Rajan Chalappurath[2*]

1 Department of Neurology, Head of Stroke Medicine Amrita Institute of Medical Sciences and Research Centre, Ernakulam, Kerala, India

2 Department of Stroke Medicine, Amrita Institute of Medical Sciences and Research Centre, Ernakulam, Kerala, India

*Address all correspondence to: drisyarajanc@gmail.com

IntechOpen

© 2019 The Author(s). Licensee IntechOpen. This chapter is distributed under the terms of the Creative Commons Attribution License (http://creativecommons.org/licenses/by/3.0), which permits unrestricted use, distribution, and reproduction in any medium, provided the original work is properly cited. (cc) BY

References

[1] Eisenhofer G, Kopin IJ, Goldstein DS. Catecholamine metabolism: A contemporary view with implications for physiology and medicine. Pharmacological Reviews. 2004;**56**:331-349

[2] Brandt M. Chapter 4: The Adrenal Medulla. In: Endocrine. Rose-Hulman Institute of Technology; pp. 49-54. Avaiable from: https://www.rosehulman.edu/~brandt/Chem330/EndocrineNotes/Chapter_4_Adrenal_Medulla.pdf

[3] Fluck DC. Catecholamines. British Heart Journal. 1972;**34**:869-873

[4] Zuber SM, Kantorovich V, Pacak K. Hypertension in pheochromocytoma: Characteristics and treatment. Endocrinology and Metabolism Clinics of North America. 2011;**40**(2):295-311

[5] Zouhal H, Jacob C, Delamarche P, Cratas A. Delamarche. Sports Medicine. 2008;**38**(5):401-423

[6] Pacak K. Pheochromocytoma: A catecholamine and oxidative stress disorder. Endocrine Regulations. 2011;**45**(2):65-90

[7] Bravo EL, Tagle R. Pheochromo-cytoma: State-of-the-art and future prospects. Endocrine Reviews. 2003;**24**(4):539-553

[8] Duka I, Gavras I, Johns C, Handy DE, Gavras H. Role of the postsynaptic α_2 adrenergic receptor subtypes in catecholamine induced vasoconstriction. General Pharmacology. 2000;**34**:101-106

[9] Giovannitti JA Jr, Thomas SM, Crawford JJ. Alpha-2 adrenergic receptor agonists: A review of current clinical applications. Anesthesia Progress. 2015;**62**(1):31-38

[10] Nedergaard OA. Catecholamines: Regulation, release and inactivation. Pharmacology and Toxicology. 1998;**1**:5-8

[11] Goldstein DS. Catecholamines and stress. Endocrine Regulations. 2003;**37**:69-80

[12] Esler MD, Hasking GJ, Willett IR, Leonard PW, Jennings GL. Noradrenaline release and SNS activity. Journal of Hypertension. 1985;**3**(2):117-129

[13] Goldstein DS, Mezey E, Yamamoto T, Aneman A, Friberg P, Eisenhofer G. Is there a third peripheral catecholaminergic system? Endogenous dopamine as an autocrine/paracrine substance derived from plasma DOPA and inactivated by conjugation. Hypertension Research. 1995;**18**:s93-s99

[14] Adameova A, Abdellaftif Y, Dhalla NS. Role of the excessive amounts of circulating catecholamines and glucocorticoids in stress-induced heart disease. Canadian Journal of Physiology and Pharmacology. 2009;**87**:493-514

[15] Wheeler MH, Chare MJB, Austin TR, Lazarus JH. The management of the patient with catecholamine excess. World Journal of Surgery. 1982;**6**:735-747

[16] Kaiser S, Chronakos J, Dietzek AM. Acute upper extremity arterial thrombosis and stroke in an unresected pheochromocytoma. Journal of Vascular Surgery. 2013;**58**(4):1069-1072

[17] Raghavan R, Ince PG, Walls TJ, Gholkar A, Dark JH, Foster JB. Malignant cerebrovascular thromboembolisation by pheochromocytoma. Clinical Neuropathology. 1995;**14**:69-71

[18] Garg SK, Garg P, Urumdas M. An interesting presentation of pheochromocytoma. Indian Journal of Critical Care Medicine. 2018;**22**(1):48-50

[19] Hou R, Leathersich AM, Rudd BT. Pheochromocytoma presenting with arterial and intracardiac thrombus in a 47-year-old woman: A case report. Journal of Medical Case Reports. 2011;**5**:310

[20] Shafiq A, Nguyen P, Hudson MP, Rabbani B. Paraganglioma as a rare cause of left ventricular thrombus in the setting of preserved ejection fraction: Discussing the literature. BML Case Reports. 2013;**2013**:1-4

[21] Wordsworth S, Thomas B, Agarwal N, Hoddell K, Davies S. Elevated urinary catecholamines and adrenal haemorrhage mimicking phaeochromocytoma. BML Case Reports. 2010;**2010**:1-3

[22] Marcasso RA, Bahr Arias MV, Gianini L, Headly SA, Bracarense APFRL. Pheochromocytoma in a dog as a cause of aortic thomboembolism. Brazilian Journal of Veterinary Pathology. 2011;**4**(2):145-149

[23] Haft JI, Kranz PD, Albert FJ, Fani K. Intravascular platelet affregation in the heart induced by norepinephrine. Circulation. 1972;**46**(4):698-708

[24] Preckel D, von Kanel R. Regulation of hemostasis by sympathetic nervous system: Any contribution to CAD? Heart. 2004;**4**(2):123-130

[25] von Kanel R, Dimsdale JE. Effects of sympathetic activation by adrenergic infusion on hemostasis in vivo. European Journal of Haematology. 2000;**65**:357-369

[26] Cimmino G, Salvatore F, Paolo G. The two faces of thrombosis: Coagulation cascade and platelet aggregation. Are platelets the main

therapeutic target? Journal of Thrombosis and Circulation: Open Access. 2017;**3**(1):117- 122

[27] Good LI, Manning AM. Thrombotic disease: Predisposition and clinical management. Compendium. 2003;**25**(9):660-675

[28] Thomas RH. Hypercoagulability syndromes. Archives of Internal Medicine. 2001;**161**:2433-2439

[29] Venugopal B, Sharon R, Abramovitz R, Khasen A, Miskin R. Plasminogen activator inhibitor-1 in cardiovascular cells: Rapid induction after injecting mice with kainath or adrenergic agents. Cardiovascular Research. 2001;**49**:476-483

[30] Cesari M, Pahor M, Incalzi RA. Plasminogen activator inhibitor-1 (PAI-1): A key factor linking fibrinolysis and age-related subclinical and clinical conditions. Cardiovascular Therapeutics. 2010;**28**(5):72-91

[31] Pickering NJ, Brody JI, Fink GB, Finnegan JO, Ablaza S. The behavior of antithombin III, alpha 2 macroglobulin and alpha 1 antitrypsin during cardiopulmonary bypass. American Journal of Clinical Pathology. 1983;**80**(4):459-464

[32] van Wersch JWJ, Rompelberg-Lahaye J, Lustermans FAT. Plasma concentration of coagulation and fibrinolysis factors and platelet function in hypertension. European Journal of Clinical Chemistry and Clinical Biochemistry. 1991;**29**:375-379

[33] van der Poll T, Levi M, Dentener M, Jansen PM, Coyle SM, Braxton CC, et al. Epinephrine exerts anticoagulant effects during human endotoxemia. The Journal of Experimental Medicine. 1997;**185**(6):1143-1148

[34] Wu KK, Thiagarajan P. Role of endothelium in thrombosis and

haemostasis. Annual Review of Medicine. 1996;**47**:315-331

[35] Gando S, Nanzaki S, Morimoto Y, Kobayashi S, Kemmotsu O. Out-of-hospital cardiac arrest increases soluble vascular endothelial adhesion molecules and neutrophil elastase associated with endothelial injury. Intensive Care Medicine. 2000;**26**:38-44

[36] Hassouna HI. Editorial comment: Blood stasis, thrombosis and fibrinolysis. Hematology/Oncology Clinics of North America. 2000;**14**(2):17-22

[37] Struyker Boudier HAJ, van Bortel LMAB, De Mey JGR. Remodelling of the vascular trace in hypertension; drug effects. Tips. 1990;**11**:240-245

[38] Ramachandran R, Rewari V. Current perioperative management of pheochromocytomas. Indian Journal of Urology. 2017;**33**(1):19

[39] Vivek K, Nambiar SS, Viswanath N, Praveen VP, Bindhu MR. Cerebral venous thrombosis due to pheochromocytoma in a patient with Von Hippel Lindau mutation. Neurology India. 2017;**65**(3):643-645

[40] Hes FJ, Hoppener JWM, Lips CJM. Pheochromocytoma in Von Hippel-Lindau disease. The Journal of Clinical Endocrinology and Metabolism. 2003;**88**(3):969-974

[41] Saposnik G, Barinagarrementeria F, Brown RD, Bushnell CD, Cucchiara B, Cushman M, et al. Diagnosis and management of cerebral venous thrombosis. Stroke. 2011;**42**:1158-1192

[42] Hiller E. Hemostatic paraneoplastic syndrome. Contributions to Oncology. 1998;**52**:122-137

[43] Semenza GL. Hydroxylation of HIF-1: Oxygen sensing at the molecular level. Physiology. 2004;**19**:176-182

[44] Semenza GL. Involvement of oxygen-sensing pathways in physiologic and pathologic erythropoiesis. Blood. 2009;**114**(10):2015-2019

[45] Jackson SP. The growing complexity of platelet aggregation. Blood. 2007;**109**(12):5087-5095. DOI: 10.1182/blood-2006-12-027698

www.ingramcontent.com/pod-product-compliance
Lightning Source LLC
Chambersburg PA
CBHW081238190326
41458CB00016B/5826